TOO SHORT A DAY
A Woman Vet in Africa

TOO SHORT A DAY

A WOMAN VET IN AFRICA

by
SUSANNE HART

TAPLINGER PUBLISHING COMPANY
NEW YORK

First published in the United States in 1967 by
TAPLINGER PUBLISHING CO. INC.
29 East Tenth Street
New York, N.Y. 10003

© SUSANNE HARTHOORN, 1966

All rights reserved. No portion of this book may be reproduced in any form without the written permission of the publisher, except by a reviewer who may wish to quote brief passages in connection with a review for a newspaper or magazine.

Library of Congress Catalog Card Number: 67-24991

PRINTED IN GREAT BRITAIN

To my patient and
loving parents—
in gratitude

Acknowledgements

Very sincere thanks are due to Hilda Stevenson-Hamilton for help and inspiration; to Howard Kirk for his wonderful companionship and for sharing so much with me, also for the photographs; to Toni Harthoorn for making it possible for me to be part of the immobilising project in the Parks and for his photographs; to my sister Alice who taught me that one must write as one speaks and thinks, spontaneously, and whose ability to laugh with me and at me helped me through many a difficult time; to faithful friends who stayed with me through thick and thin and who never let me give up: Athalie Waugh, Angela van Royen, Bobbie Papas, Valerie and Esias Bosch; and last, but not least, my grateful thanks to Mr Jock Gibb, my publisher, who encouraged me to persevere.

S. H.

Contents

Chapter		Page
	INTRODUCTION	13
1.	EARLY DAYS	15
2.	TOUCH OF THE VET	23
3.	RETURN TO PRACTICE	34
4.	OF LIONS, ELEPHANTS AND PYTHONS	47
5.	THE RELUCTANT BULL	58
6.	EVEN A MOUSE...	67
7.	ZEBRA IN THE MIST	79
8.	FAMOUS PEOPLE AND JUNGLE ADDICTS	91
9.	SONGOLOLO IN MY BED	109
10.	CAESARIAN IN THE SUN	124
11.	THE POTTER'S HAND	138
12.	BOTTLES ON MY SHELF	149
13.	VULTURES' PARADISE	161
14.	GONZO THE GIANT	168
15.	RIDE A WILD RHINO	179

Key to photographers

a   Bill Sinclair
b   Howard Kirk
c   Puck Brinkman
d   The author
e   Terence Reilly
f   Hilda Stevenson-Hamilton
g   A. M. Harthoorn
h   B. Chappell
i   Harold Weaver

Illustrations

1. The author and her microscope[a]   *facing page* 48
2. Herd sentry[b]   49
3. The author's children with their pets[c]   49
4. Chico[b]   64
5. Hyenas[b]   64
6. Joâo[d]   65
7. Twinkletoes[b]   80
8. Lulu[e]   80
9. "Skukusa"[f]   81
10. Hilda Stevenson-Hamilton[b]   81
11. Immobilised zebra[g]   96
12. Immobilised elephant[h]   96
13. Immobilised giraffe[g]   97
14. A baboon[b]   112
15. Everyone was used to this Yoga exercise[g]   113
16. Toni Harthoorn[g]   128
17. The author's sister with her two children[i]   128
18. The author performing surgery[a]   129
19. The author and Sam with Lucky and Cheetah[g]   129
20. The author's dog "Ricci". *From a painting by Theo Papas*   160
21. Esias Bosch[g]   160
22. A chameleon stripping off its skin[b]   161
23. Vultures feeding[b]   161
24. The author and Howard Kirk treating an owl[a]   176
25. The author astride a wild white rhino[g]   177
26. John Clarke with a white rhino[g]   177

(For photographers see opposite)

Introduction

Seven years ago, these hills and forests where I have made my home seemed very far away. As I listened to my well-meaning friends, the jagged rocks and mountain-tops became positively menacing, and I could almost imagine the burning heat and the never-ceasing summer floods. "You would be mad to put one foot into that jungle country," they admonished, "a woman alone with two small children. You have no experience whatsoever of the wild beasts that roam there nor have you ever worked among such a population of farmers, with the reputation of being equally wild. The Lowveld is unhealthy and primitive; you would not last more than six months, and if you did, you would become a shrivelled, tired shadow of your former self."

This conjured up a frightening vision of myself, pickled in formalin (veterinary style) in a jar on the shelf for all to see and point at and say: "There floats the woman vet who would not listen to good advice!" Their words, spoken in the spirit of protectiveness, nevertheless did not deter me. The whole country lay open to me, yet it was in this lovely jungle that I chose to live. I did not do this in a spirit of female perversity, but simply because the Lowveld had already cast its magic upon me previously when, for a short year, I had lived among those peaceful purple hills, whose beauty is at once gentle and violently African.

Working and living among these people, from the high alpine Sabie mountains to the hot low-lying and sweet-scented citrus lands, has been – and is – a wonderful experience. It is as though an enchantment radiates from every stick and stone and bird; there is a continuity running through the changes of seasons and the fall of night. The slow rhythm of life is not a lazy pace, for here the farmers produce some of the loveliest fruit and vegetables and straightest, strongest timber in the Republic.

Times are harder and leaner than they were when I first came, and the prosperity of the Lowveld has become a memory. But there must always be an ebb and flow in the affairs of men, and so I believe that the Wheel of Fortune will turn, bringing better times once again.

As I write, this paradisial country clings to the last skirts of winter, and soon the sun-baked land will once again grow green with the coming of the summer's rains. But now the atmosphere is charged with electricity, the extreme dryness makes one feel skin-tight and tense. Yet even in this hot time of breathless waiting for the sight of rain clouds in the sky, the countryside glows with deep red and purple and yellow. It is wonderful how these blooms and shrubs are nourished; in my dry garden, which I dare not water now, the Cup of Gold has a bell-like resonance of colour and the texture of silk. The birds are in a spring fever, each seeking a mate and a place to nest. Their splendour both of voice and plumage are still daily wonders to me.

All this is the backdrop of my work. Because of this I am here; and there is plenty to do, since Nature not only gives but also takes away some of her gifts. This is one of the most disease-ridden parts of South Africa: it draws to itself not only man, but also every pest and parasite, visible and invisible; disease of plant and tree and beast often remains an unsolved riddle, but those who suffer from the resultant losses seem to be strengthened and fortified by the very atmosphere of their environment. Struggling against great odds, they fight to remain on their own soil in their beloved Lowveld, preferring to live humbly rather than forsake their way of life.

CHAPTER 1

Early Days

If the signs of the Zodiac control our characters, it is small wonder that I should choose a veterinary career. I was born under Taurus the bull, and named after a dog: yet my parents still wonder how it came about that I chose this unladylike profession. My earliest memories of delirious happiness are connected with the smell of cow dung, the rough texture of calf tongues, and the frothy sound of milk flowing into the pail in a steady streaming rhythm.

I was a problem child: not only did I turn out a girl instead of a boy, but I was also in a constant state of rebellion. I only wanted one thing, to live in the country; yet I was born into a family of city dwellers. My father and mother were very tolerant and loving, but they found my attitude incomprehensible, since there were no rural precedents in our family, nor had I had any remote contact with the country *in utero*.

Once out of the city I was lost to them. The nearer I could get to the good earth, the happier I was. My poor mother lived in terror of all cows and bulls, though I think she hardly knew the difference between them. To see me disappear among these ominous beasts early in the morning, and to have to haul me out at mealtimes, must have caused her unspeakable horror. She was always scrubbing, disinfecting and admonishing me. I sought the companionship of farm-hands and milkmaids, preferred climbing trees to doing embroidery, and excelled in fist-fights and other boyish pastimes.

When I was five we were summering in the Austrian Alps; every pair of hands was employed in bringing in the harvest. This was absolute bliss for me, since I was allowed to go out into the fields, sharing the cider and oatcakes at midday, revelling in the company of the happy and boisterous workers.

It was on such a day that my fate was decided. A small fieldmouse was injured by a worker's scythe, and I managed to rescue the little creature before the *coup de grace* was delivered. Ignoring the cries of my companions, I ran back to the farm-house as fast as my short legs could carry me, burst into my mother's room, and, before she had time to recover from her surprise, I poured the entire contents of her eau-de-Cologne bottle (specially imported from Paris) over the body of the suffering victim, certain that any broken or injured limbs would be immediately healed by such a potent liquid. My mother was much more reasonable about the whole affair than one might have expected, and even lent me her soft handkerchief so that I might wrap up the little bundle and keep it warm. She comforted me when my patient died some hours later, showing great love and understanding coupled with a compassion for my own agony which entirely overcame her own disapproval of my behaviour. I buried the corpse in a flowerpot, and for days my poor parents suffered from the smell: at last, overcome by conscience, I confessed my sin and removed what was left to the soil under the big shady cherry-tree.

This small incident was the beginning of my veterinary career. After that, my purpose in life became clear and I systematically began to collect animal waifs and strays, taking them home for love, food and care. My parents suffered these flea-bitten mongrels with patience, knowing that my happiness depended on their own tolerance. Secretly they hoped that I would grow out of this phase, and attempted to turn my thoughts to other careers. They did not at any time decrease their efforts to turn me from a tomboy into a lady; and have never told me, to this day, whether they feel they have succeeded in this task.

After leaving school at the age of sixteen, and before entering the Royal Veterinary College, I spent a long vacation near Bedford, learning the art of farming from three delightful maiden ladies. They reared all types of stock with a love and dedication that I never imagined possible. It was a farm of individualists; the collie dog rounded up the cattle at milking time without the help of anyone, the pony I drove took me to the village and showed me the way. This pony also had the curious habit of stopping for a few minutes at each pub we passed, and could not be persuaded to continue at any cost; I discovered afterwards that its previous owner had been a vet!

I learnt how to rear squealing baby pigs on the bottle and how to call each of two hundred sheep by name; how to harness the plough-horse and how to encourage him with respectable swear-words.

I became accustomed to working my way each morning through a huge bowl of stiff and salted oatmeal porridge, and finally overcame my tendency to feel afterwards that a concrete-like lump had settled permanently in my stomach.

The only human male on the farm was the young and handsome nephew of my hostesses, a little older than myself, but not yet seventeen. I immediately fell in love with him and he with me; our tryst was sealed with a hen-ring which he stole from one of the roosters, and which we thought looked magnificent on my engagement finger. When my face became horribly distorted with itchy red sores a few days later, we realised that the source of this scourge lay in the ring, for it turned out to be 'red mite', burrowing under the skin, and very bad for my inflated ego and my vanity. In spite of this unfortunate end to my first engagement I still relish the memory of the incident, and I feel sure that we were the only couple who ever became engaged in such a rustic and original manner.

This was my launching into university, the transition period between the sheltered life of boarding-school and the world of student life, where there was no shelter and no protection. This new and carefree existence went to my head like champagne, and I played my way through first year, tasting the delights which the adult world had to offer. Lectures were dull, amounting to periods of dictation, but even so those days were very gay. The examiners were kind and let some errants through, though many others failed before the course was over. Out of one hundred and ten in our first year, ten were girls; we ended up sixty in our final year, including six girls, 'survivors' in a real sense, since we had much to endure from our fellow students, and were not entirely welcome in the college. These were the post-war years, when ex-servicemen were waiting to come back to continue their studies; we were always regarded as husband-seekers rather than as serious-minded vets, and our places were naturally coveted. But this was little more than a mood: we even got some preferential treatment. By our second year, we 'ladies' were not quite so much ostracised, and were even allowed to listen to the incredibly smutty stories which

B

are a tradition among all medical students. This was indeed an honour, but I must confess that most of these stories went completely over my head.

At that age I hardly understood the facts of life, and was very immature compared with many of my companions; I thought that I would simply continue my tomboyish type of life at college. I felt very strongly on the subject of equality of the sexes; I saw no reason why, as a female student, I could not simply continue as before, moulding myself into the veterinary way of life, becoming part of the student mass and remaining sexless, or if anything retaining my boyish character. These illusions were shattered almost at once on entering the University. The first function of the year, and a tradition at the R.V.C., was the so-called 'heifer sale' dance, where the freshettes were simply lined up and appraised like young bovines, being subjected to the indignity of minute and thorough top-to-toe examination by the seasoned veterans, the senior students. For the first time in my life I was made to feel like a second-class citizen in a world of men; worse than that, I was made to feel female to the point of embarrassment.

This significant event put me thoroughly in my place. Having longed to be part of the world of men, I now slowly came to understand that, having been endowed with a female figure and personality for no obvious reason, I must face facts and settle down to make the best of things. Having reached this decision, life became easier. From now on, I simply had to prove that I could hold my own as a woman, and meanwhile learn the subtleties and arts which enable us to hold our sway without man being aware of it. I contented myself with gaining honours as a poker player, satisfied to be accepted as an equal there if nowhere else.

Some of our teachers saw the necessity of giving us guidance, and took us under their wing before we had gone too far. In spite of their long hours of work and their research activities they gave us freely of their time; they tolerated our inadequacies, gave us courage at examination-time, listened to our problems, even helped us to sort out our love affairs.

One aspect of our studies held particular fascination for me. This was microscopy, the study in minute detail of the fantastic composition and structure of the cell, healthy and diseased. After lectures, some of us would sometimes be permitted to remain behind and witness the amazing activities of the dividing ovum under the microscope. Professor Amoroso, who encouraged this, had such enthusiasm for his work that the whole process of learning embryology became a wonderful and exciting adventure.

In the late afternoon we would all adjourn to an old pub near by and share tankard after tankard of beer, while the conversation turned from science to more suitable and light-hearted subjects: we relaxed in the smoke-laden atmosphere, student and teacher on equal terms; everything was thrashed out at such times, from the underworld life of London to the chemistry of love. My narrow horizons were much widened on those occasions; the cobwebs of the secluded years gradually fell away and I matured, without being aware of it.

During the two years I spent in London, my family home was subjected to disorder and chaos, for veterinary students are usually rowdy and animal in their ways. I shared a room with my kind and gentle sister, who did not delight in the rows of pickled creatures decorating the desk, or in the smell of formalin and methylated spirits which clung to the entire contents of the room from curtains to underwear. She only complained when I hid decapitated frogs in her bed, knowing well her horror of all creepy-crawly things. Veterinary students are somehow different from others, easily recognisable even when they are dressed neatly, which rarely happens.

My sister became a very good diagnostician of the type, insisting that about us clings for ever an aroma composed chiefly of mice, horse-manure, dissection rooms and beer. It is much to her credit that in spite of this she readily associated with my friends, and even retained her love for her eccentric sister.

These were, indeed, days of great trial for my parents. I don't think they knew whether they preferred the flea-infested mongrels of my childhood days or the wild, unkempt human companions of my later years. Coming home with the milk after wild student orgies, disrupting their gentle-flowing Mozart symphony with blasts upon the hunting-horn when my escorts called for me – such things did little to maintain a harmonious family relationship. I suspect that when I departed for the country field station in my fourth year of college, my family was just a little glad to see some distance put between us.

London days were over, and so were the days of endless taking of notes, endless late nights, and the confusion that students suffer when let loose in a big city. It marked a new phase of college life, for once the third year is left behind one is well on the way to becoming a vet. We, of course, already considered ourselves as vets, being at an age when we were not overcome by either modesty or humility!

Country life for me meant freedom. The Thames Valley between Reading and Oxford was the setting for our last two college years, and it would have been impossible to choose a more beautiful part of England: the green undulating hills, gently following the curves of the river, have a unique beauty. Although no more easily than in the city, we could study more profitably in the clean untainted air: there was very little to distract us, apart from the glorious pubs, and the work at last took on a practical nature, so that we felt in touch with the purpose of our study.

A dear but slightly impoverished lady let the upper story of her house to a group of us; this became our digs, and a place also where male students could get a reasonable meal for the price of chopping a load of wood.

Those two years whipped past us with lightning speed. We walked a great deal, rode along the green hill-tops (known as the Fairmile) where race-horses are trained, we sailed, climbed, went to Oxford and to Reading for our amusements, and studied a great deal more than we had in London. It was in vacation-time that we did most of our work, for we spent five months of our annual 'holidays' working with veterinary practitioners.

We worked very hard doing our 'practice'. The college had a list of eminent veterinarians who agreed to take us on, and from these we got a very good taste of veterinary work. We had to present a series of case records at our final examinations, signed and approved, and this forced us to take particular and detailed notes of our holiday work, and to follow up the cases by post even after we had returned to college. To me this was genuine learning; at the time I rather rebelled against bookwork, and disliked having to memorise facts I felt sure I would never need again.

I learned much from a woman vet who, although she appeared

very mannish, had the kindest and gentlest manner with animals, and who excelled at all practice, large and small. In action, her illusion of maleness immediately disappeared, for no man could ever have the sensitivity, kindness and patience that this woman – at the top of her profession – possessed.

I have seen her perform miracles of healing through perserverance, when most people would have given up. She had the most wonderful approach; she did not proceed to treat, or even to examine, until she had made definite contact with her patients; and she did not mind how long this took, even on a busy day. She was curt and to the point with people, but with animals she took great pains to establish contact, and in some way she usually did succeed, with even the most hostile. From her I also learnt much of the history of woman vets in England: they were now established as part and parcel of the profession, but in her days woman students were treated as outcasts. The first woman veterinary student in London who dared to wear slacks was duly de-panted, and her trousers hoisted on the college chimney. Women students were regarded as curiosities, and this attitude survived vestigially into my own student days.

It was, however, another woman veterinary surgeon who nearly broke down my desire to continue with my studies. She was a younger person, and seemed quite devoid of any feelings for her patients. I was extremely unhappy with her, and the final blow came when we went to destroy a large and very old dog. It was the first destruction I had ever witnessed. The lady vet simply threw some prussic acid into the eye of the dog, whereupon he went into the most ghastly and severe convulsions. I was too shocked to speak, but my face must have made my feelings clear, for she tried to justify her behaviour. Her point was clear; it was cheaper to use prussic acid, and as the dog had to die in any case, why waste time and money on the intravenous method?

When she mentioned speed I saw red. Who can judge the length of the last seconds of life? And who are we, already in the wrong by taking life so often and so needlessly, to try and judge and justify ourselves? Drowning men, who have recovered, have said that in those seconds when the life-force was running out their whole lives were reviewed before them. Whatever the truth of it was, I was ready to leave this practice and the veterinary career altogether.

In later years this nightmare experience came back to me time and time again. It came as a warning, and incentive for greater patience and understanding, and it made me delve very deeply into the question of different methods of destruction; finally, it made me realise that when we take it upon ourselves to snuff out lives, we often have no right to do so, any more than the doctor has the right to terminate a human life.

CHAPTER 2

Touch of the Vet

"Please Miss, come out to my farm, my chickens are losing all their feathers." I was doing locum, my first ever, at the age of nineteen, a raw student shaking at the knees, with so little knowledge that the harassed chicken farmer would have preferred to let a few more feathers fall out rather than call me, had she known.

In those days we were often pitched at the unsuspecting public to get some practical training (in the capacity of locum tenens) before we had qualified. This was a marvellous way to gain confidence and experience, and it gave the always overworked veterinarian a chance to get a holiday. Usually and wisely, they remained within phoning distance, but not on this bright and sunny morning. All of a sudden it was not bright and sunny any more. The whole world seemed to be one mass of chickens in a fix, and the breeze blew feathers everywhere. I was in a dither, to put it mildly; I racked my brain, but no inspiration came; I searched the books, but of course in my haste could not find anything of any use. The phone rang again. "Dear Miss, please do not be too long, I am sure the chickens will catch cold!" Dear God, what next?

Into the little car. I had only a learner's licence and had twice failed my test in London. Any traffic policeman would have *heard* a mile off that I was a shocking driver, just by the way I grated the gears! The little Austin was so ancient and student-battered that nothing I could do would damage it further. I reached the farm, said silent prayers to the dear Lord to be specially kind to a poor student vet and plunged headlong into my first case.

The chickens, White Leghorns of the most aristocratic variety, looked appalling. The lady who owned them looked worse, in spite of the fact that she wore more protective clothing than they.

I made a start in the most professional manner I could muster; I spent an hour examining and asking questions, my mind all the while murmuring a silent supplication. "Yes," I suddenly found myself saying, "there is only one thing to do. Crush the egg-shells and feed them back. The feathers will soon grow again." And they did!

After one week the lady phoned me in ecstasy; I had become the heroine of the local chicken industry, my powers were miraculous. All the feathers were growing again after two weeks. I was delighted, but could take no credit; I wondered and wondered from what corner of my slow-functioning, not-retentive brain this vital information had suddenly trickled in upon my consciousness.

It was also upon a fowl that I performed my first piece of unaided surgery. This particular hen was crop-bound; I had heard it said that there is very little sensation in the superficial skin of poultry and birds, but the thought of attempting a literal vivisection filled me with horror. At last I resolved to try, and very gently and slowly I opened up the crop, and to my amazement there was no reaction whatsoever from my patient. With triumph in my heart I emptied the overfull sack, and having washed it, began to sew up the wound with clumsy and inexperienced fingers, intent upon each stitch and each knot, trying hard not to create 'granny' knots, the worst a veterinary seamstress can produce. I was so absorbed in my task that I did not at first notice that the little hen was also extremely busy; she was, in fact, pecking up again what I had just removed from her crop, as fast as she could, and I wondered if I would have to start the operation all over again. This finally brought home the truth of my colleagues' contention, that we must never waste our good local anaesthetic solution on a mere bird.

My student days become more vivid to me as time goes on. All this happened sixteen years ago, yet the pattern of those days is very detailed. The same kind of people and animals seems always to recur; then as now, I often wondered whether the seven human types, astrologically classified, can also be detected in the animal kingdom. And the sensation of having seen and heard someone before, is a striking and familiar one.

The day I began to write this chapter, I was strongly reminded of a long-ago incident. A golden spaniel was brought into my room; he was exactly like one that had been brought into the surgery in my student-practice days, becoming an object of much comment. I had just returned from the lunch-break, and on my way to join my senior in the office, I noticed a golden Cocker tied to the table-leg in the dressing-room. Wondering why he was there, for he looked sleek and well, I approached him and spent some happy moments playing with him. As I was about to untie him a voice called out to me: "What ever you do, Sue, don't touch the yellow monster in the back room. He has just bitten another child and has to be destroyed." I could hardly believe it. I turned back to the dog, this time with my mind in a different state: he smelled my sudden suspicion and fear, subconscious though it was, and would not allow me to approach him. From a soft and gentle creature, he had turned into a snarling horror in a matter of a few moments; an incredible change, and I was profoundly shocked. I realised then that the receptive apparatus of the dog is like the finest radar station imaginable. The signals he had received from me in those seconds had impressed themselves upon his highly-developed super-sensory organs, probably both telepathically and by means of the scent-receivers, or perhaps the lightning speed of the reaction was due to a combination of both. It is possible that this highly-bred type of dog is more receptive than an easy-going mongrel or less over-bred type.

In the years of practice, I have observed many similar cases, and have myself probably developed some kind of protective shell which will not allow any fear to communicate itself to my patients too easily. There has never been a vet who is completely devoid of fear, even as an uncontrolled sensation; but if this fear breaks through one might as well give up the veterinary career, for I believe that most species respond to human attitudes not only in their own behaviour but in their response to treatment as well. A veterinary practitioner has not only the task of curing the 'outside' animal; he also has to instil confidence and peace of mind into his patient, just as the human doctor does with his.

It was during my student-practice days that I discovered something about life and about people which many fail to learn until much later. I lived with the poor and the rich while in digs, and I was able to study them, and sometimes live through their heartaches with them. The importance to the vet of the owner-animal relationship was made clear to me as I discovered why people keep animals: economics, sentiment, necessity, these were the three things I found. Now that I have practised for some years, I would add convention and habit.

Farming economically and sometimes scientifically can be a great joy. Some farmers do it decently, not only weighing the value on the hoof or in the udder, but also weighing up the needs and souls of the animals that serve them. They farm with dignity and kindness, and they suffer a little when their beasts have to go to market. The second type farms meanly, to make as much out of his stock as he can, putting in as little as possible. He is a menace to all vets, for he calls for help too late, and begrudges payment. Such a man has no right to farm with animals at all; he should stick to the inanimate and the mechanised.

What a greenhorn I was! I thought that everyone farmed for sentiment: to see their herds grazing, or the strength and beauty of their plough-horses at work. When I was among farmers in the North of England, this illusion crashed about my ears; here people were needy, and a little hardened in consequence. They cursed and kicked their animals, who flinched therefore when one approached them. I learnt about that kind of life the hard way, and it was one of the most useful lessons I ever learnt. It seems a pity that human-animal relationships are not taught as a special subject in college, for they are a vital part of our life.

While up north I often worked with the local vet, and one day I went with him to treat a cow. She was very ill, and the treatment would take weeks. The vet examined her – examined the owner also, I noticed – and advised immediate destruction. I was appalled and condemned him utterly in my own mind; yet I was confused, for he was a kindly man. Only much later, when I dared to question him did the truth come out. "They will never look after her or nurse her," he said, "better for all concerned that she die at once and mercifully than a slow and painful death. They will never call me in to see her again! Don't let it get you down," he added, "our duty is to do our best and act correctly and in the most humane manner. If you take every case home with you for supper you will live a life of heartbreak." He was absolutely right, but unfortunately, perhaps because I am a woman, I could not carry out his advice to the letter. Perhaps it is better to suffer a little after all; perhaps it enables one to see more deeply into the suffering of others.

My parents allowed me to visit Denmark during my eighteenth year. This was to prove the experience of a lifetime for me, for not only was the Copenhagen veterinary institution very progressive, but it was crowded with the largest collection of devastatingly handsome men I have ever seen in my life. I went during the long summer vacation, and stayed with good friends, who did everything to make my stay an unforgettable one. Apart from the work, I was taken to see much of the picturesque countryside, and was amazed to find how harmoniously a nationalised country functions. Admittedly it is a pocket-size nation of only four million people, but it does seem that the temperament of the inhabitants is conducive to the smooth running of such a community. The Danes are an equable, kind, broadminded people, and I was relieved to find that everyone, from bus drivers to school children, could speak English well enough to make my life there a very easy one. Too easy, perhaps, for the only way to learn a foreign tongue is to live among the people. I did struggle to assimilate a small vocabulary, but Danish is an extremely difficult language and quite unlike the ones I had some knowledge of, such as French and German. As I entered a lecture hall the lecturer would immediately switch from Danish to English in the most effortless manner, thus enabling me to make full use of their excellent course.

It occurred to me to do my final year in the Copenhagen Veterinary School. The method of examination appealed to me immensely, as it excluded our most barbaric end-of-the-year agonies. In Denmark the whole year's work is taken into consideration, practically and theoretically. The heads of departments are wholly responsible for the weighing up of each student's worth, and at the end of each year oral examinations only are carried out, not by some stranger from outside, but by each student's own familiar teacher. This is a wonderful and humane system and should be adopted everywhere. At our own examinations (which lasted for days and days, during which time we got progressively more tense and haggard) outside examiners were called in who often had little contact with the teaching of the particular subject or with students in general. In our final year a famous and respected gentleman came to examine us in surgery. Although he had been a great authority on horse-practice in his time (about thirty years back), this battered and unspeakably aged veteran was almost entirely deaf, and was unfortunately possessed of the fiercest taste in cruel humour. He hardly understood our answers, even when we shouted them into his ear for the third time; then he would assure us gruffly that we were entirely and hopelessly wrong, that our standard was low and our knowledge inadequate. He would choose the exact psychological moment, when the student was off guard and in the last stage of examination fever, to ask a ludicrous question of which we had been warned: "What does the horse break when it falls at the fence?" Most wise and apprehensive students hesitated before they answered, and this often saved them. "Well, what did you say?" he would bellow, and if the victim gave the correct answer he would look positively disappointed.

However, many a student had by this time fallen into a sort of stupor, and like a quivering bird hypnotised by a hissing snake, simply had to give the wrong answer, in spite of himself. That was the end, and no reprieve. Since anatomy days we had known that a cat and a horse are constructed without a collar bone: a cat so as to squeeze through narrow chinks, and a horse so as to trip up students. This slip-up, whatever the conditions, meant failure in the subject and therefore in the whole year, surgery being of vital importance.

There was however, a lighter side to all this, and many stories were told about incidents which did much to dispel the examination-time tension. One young lady, having been asked how she would proceed at the onset of a calving case, immediately began to strip down to the waist, demonstrating that anything that male vets could do, she could do too. The examiner was beside himself with alarm that this might be misconstrued were anyone else to arrive on the scene! On another occasion a lady student was required to examine the udder of a cow for mastitis, and in placing her hand on the relevant place found the examiner's hand and held it – hopeful, perhaps, that this might give her preferential treatment. Having completed her task, she coyly inquired how the learned gentleman liked her work, and received the reply: "I like it so much that you will just have to come back next year and do it all over again!"

What could be more unfair? On top of this torture, the woman students were repeatedly warned not to wear silk stockings (this was before the days of nylon plenty) or make-up, and to look as unattractive as possible. Failure to appear thus would spell certain displeasure with the worst possible consequences. The result was utterly demoralising, for not only did we need more make-up, to hide the dark shadows and pallid skin acquired during weeks of too many books and too little sunlight, but the male students were appalled by our appearance at a time when they needed extra cheer. Apparently the archaic school of examiners were all against sex-appeal; in spite of their disapproval we had been permitted to take the veterinary course, but they would at least see to it that no vamping was done during examinations. I suppose in a way this was a compliment to our feminity, and their fear was partly justified by the fact that most of the female students passed the first two years, when little serious work was done, by sex-appeal and little else.

Small wonder that I longed to escape this fate! But as the veterinary degree in Denmark is of less value in Britain than the English one, I abandoned my scheme and returned home.

The following long vacation I spent in France, not on the Riviera, but working with a vet among the people of the mountains, in Auvergne. This was thought up by the 'interchange of students' scheme, a marvellous system filled with the promise of adventure. The prospect of my going into a strange country among strange people filled my parents with apprehension. They knew France well enough to realise that a girl of nineteen with a complete trust in humanity and little common sense took quite a chance in going there. They warned me endlessly about the many dangers which might confront me; particularly the water, which they said was practically undrinkable due to bad hygiene. The more they worried, the happier I became, hoping against hope that all their fears were justified, being impatient at the slow passage of time before my departure.

I was met at the Gare du Nord by Jean, the son of M. Guichard, who was a veterinary student at Alfort, outside Paris. We had previously sent each other exact descriptions so as to obviate any confusion at the station, which was milling with colourful and deafening humanity. I gathered my belongings, and waited, and waited. There were many others doing the same thing; surely they were not all there to meet someone they had never seen before?

After an hour, when I was just about in tears, a small bespectacled man approached me, hesitantly flourishing a letter. "It surely cannot be you, *vous êtes si belle!*" What an overstatement, for I was travel- and tear-stained, bedraggled, hot, and at the end of my tether. He explained that he had not dared to approach me, since from my own description of myself, "tall and dark and thin", he had gathered a different impression, and in any case a potential vet-ess should (he felt) look like a cross between a goat and a cow. Perhaps I misunderstood him, my French was very weak at the time.

We became the best of friends, and for a few days I stayed in digs near Alfort while he showed me the city in true student fashion. This was the only way of getting to know Paris; student haunts, the less expensive joys, the real Paris, not the tourist variety. I ate horse-meat, drank wine – sparingly at first but quickly increasing my daily intake after a telegram had arrived from my dear and ever-worrying mother: "Remember, whatever you do, do not drink the French water." I obeyed her. I drank wine at least six times a day, whenever I was thirsty. The result was that my French improved tremendously and any remnant of my mother's other warnings sank into oblivion. The wine also lessened the shock of my first contact with bed-bugs, and I felt so exhilarated that I could bear my landlady no grudge when normally such bed-companions would have sent me packing.

I enjoyed myself enormously and my harassed parents got only a hastily scribbled postcard on which I briefly mentioned that I loved Frenchmen, had unusual bed-companions, and promised never to drink water again. As a result they phoned all the way to Haute-Loire, the little village where Jean's father worked, and spoke long and threateningly across the channel. My host reassured them in his best English, which was limited to an amusing version of "To be or not to be" and to some five or six other words besides. Whatever he said obviously had the right effect, for there were no more urgent trans-Channel calls thereafter.

It was a hauntingly lovely section of France, as poor as it was lovely. The family had conducted a fine practice in Paris until the war, and then moved south to this forgotten never-never land, to work and to assist the French Underground. After the war they had stayed on, living in a narrow three-storeyed house without sewerage and with little home comfort, but surrounded by magnificent views and by warm-hearted and loyal people. Practice here was something of a revelation, for the communities, mainly clumped together on mountain heights, lived under appalling conditions, were riddled with tuberculosis, and diseases which are the result of inbreeding. Their stock was unhealthy, uneconomical and depleted.

Everywhere the contrasts were striking. The churches, built on the topmost peaks, were constructed of stone and possessed an almost unearthly beauty. The inhabitants were intensely religious and entirely Catholic, and to them their church was life itself as well as a symbol of life. The countryside was filled with wild cherries, sweet-scented cyclamen, strawberries, mushrooms, and forests of ancient pine, untapped and unused. The streams were crowded with fish, the meadows with wild flowers. A paradise for vagabonds, for one could live on what nature provided alone. Yet poverty was everywhere, and with it went a generous and kind, carefree spirit of companionship, quite unlike anything I had found in poor country in England.

I was made welcome and became one with these people; I learnt to speak the language their way, fish their way, eat and drink their way. For the first week I was somewhat muzzy, since each job of work we did was followed by a family social hour round the kitchen table, drinking the home-brewed beverages which were more than a little alcoholic. Gradually I became accustomed to my new mode of life, and felt so much part of the Guichard family that I could not bear the thought of leaving. Their frank approach to life, their openness in matters of sex was a little staggering for an inexperienced freshette. Jean, a charming but ardent boy of twenty, found me just as puzzling and often laughingly referred to me as "de frigide English miss".

I learnt how to eat *écrevisses*, prepared in boiling oil; and how to cleanse a cow of its retained afterbirth. It was thus that I also caught Undulant Fever, as it was diagnosed when I returned to

London, making rather an antibiotic anticlimax to my French adventure. Nevertheless, developing an occupational disease so early on in my career made me feel rather superior; I almost felt that this was a preliminary qualification for my veterinary degree.

My parents had just returned from a glorious orgy of music in Edinburgh, and they were very relieved to see me home in one piece, with no other damage than a Brucella infection.

It was good to travel. However little I assimilated, it did much to assuage my wanderlust; and to know how others work and live is a humbling experience. It sets one's own life into perspective, before one grows into too big a balloon of self-worship and consequently has the longer way to fall when the ego becomes deflated. All students need this; nor does it end there. We need it all our working lives, for a veterinarian is a very important part of the community, not for animal attendance alone but because he is often the person to whom the lady of the house confesses her inmost secrets about her husband, her neighbours, her fears and her joys. It seems strange that a vet should invite these confidences even more than a doctor; perhaps it is because most of us have a free-and-easy manner which comes from dealing with uncomplicated creatures like cows and white mice, rather than with neurotic patients who call a doctor for anything from an itchy toe to an overfilled stomach.

Working close to the land puts one at ease. A country vet usually is a roaming, happy person; the variety, the manner of life make him an easy companion. He is lost without a good sense of humour, for his patience is tried more than an ordinary doctor's. Many a time will he arrive at a farm, to find the patient returned to pasture; this may mean a long wait and a little less leisure and peace at the end of the day, but nevertheless he must not become ruffled; he must be philosophical and sit and sip his coffee and make small talk. Sometimes I have suspected that this sort of delay is purposely arranged so that the lady of the house may get some problem off her chest! One very handsome veterinarian in London with whom I practised was often called to attend to ladies' pets who were obviously in the best of health. I was not made to feel particularly welcome at these times, but the long-suffering practitioner used to console me with a broad wink, and make a great show of trying to find the non-existent cause of a non-existent ailment.

My Professor in Surgery rendered me a great kindness by quietly and unofficially telling me I had passed the final year examinations, thus releasing me from the anxiety of waiting and wondering. He mentioned the possibility of a post for me, which offered good scope and wages; and he was much saddened when I told him that I was engaged to be married to a South African, and would be sailing within two weeks. It was by no means an easy thing to tell him, for I knew his thoughts on the subject; all those years of study wasted; those overcrowded colleges, with far more applications than places. Yes, I knew exactly what was running through his mind: I was another failure, another reason for barring women students from the veterinary course. I hung my head in shame and left: I could not bear to see the disappointment in his eyes. My mind was wholly occupied with the glamour of my forthcoming marriage, with travel to new lands, new people. I had no conception then, that I would ever practise my vocation, or that my marriage would not be a permanent career. My parents did not mind; only my happiness, in whatever manner of life I chose, had any importance to them.

CHAPTER 3

Return to Practice

Five years later I was living in Port Elizabeth expecting my second child. Veterinary practice seemed a thing of far away and long ago, and as time passed my interest lessened to a point where I barely glanced at the veterinary journals which I still continued to receive. My life was fully occupied, and I spent my days doing the sort of things all women do, with the additional joy of daily sea-swimming in one of the quiet unfrequented pools which abound on that part of the coast.

One afternoon, while I was vegetating lazily in the garden, a car pulled up outside the gate and a tall, pink-complexioned man came sauntering across the lawn. His manner was informal and easy, hardly that of a stranger, yet I was certain I had not met him before. He smiled at my puzzlement, lowered himself into the chair next to mine, and gazed at me speculatively as though he was assessing my condition (which he was). "Dovey is the name: John Dovey. Heard last week that there is a female colleague in the vicinity; no one told me that you are in calf."

How like a vet! Straight to the point, no fuss, the healthy unsophisticated approach of a man used to working with animals. Suddenly I was hungry to hear about veterinary practice and longed for the sweet aroma of a surgery, the Dettol–ether–methylated spirit smell which was once like magic to me. John must have realised how I felt and nodded his head in approval. "When you have calved down," he said nonchalantly, "come and watch around for the odd morning, see how you feel. Maybe your veterinary days are not over yet."

The following month I duly bore my son, Guy David. My veterinary friend dropped in to see me whenever he was in the area, bringing me news of his world, giving me the incentive and some of his enthusiasm. When my baby was a few months old and sleeping through the mornings, I took my courage in both my hands and slipped out and up the hill to see if I really still had an interest in my chosen career. White-coated and professional, Doctor Dovey met me as I walked in, and before I could blink an eyelid or entertain a single doubt he addressed me: "Oh, there you are, please come in and give me your opinion on this case." He certainly had the knack of breaking the professional ice; before I knew it I was actually giving an opinion.

This was the beginning. I often slipped out in the morning and snatched a few hours doing the work that I found I still loved. I was unpractised and clumsy, but little by little the feeling of it came back and my self-confidence grew. Then one day John declared that he badly needed a few days' holiday and hoped to leave in three days. Would I please do him the favour of helping him to avert a threatened ulcer by doing his work? How could I refuse? I set about organising my family and waved the overworked vet good-bye at the docks. Deep down I always knew that he went away to give me the chance to work alone – the only way for me to regain confidence and get on my veterinary feet again.

I really was alone. Seven days have never contained so many hours before, nor has any hour contained so many minutes. It was a busy week, crowned by a Caesarian section on a dying cat. To everyone's amazement the poor creature recovered, strengthened perhaps by the patron saint of vets who must have stood over us with his magic wand. It was nothing short of a miracle, a definite landmark in my veterinary career. I had the continued moral support of Daphne, John Dovey's wife, who cheered me on throughout my days of trial and consoled me when things did not go smoothly.

By the time my friend and mentor returned I was altogether a different girl, and very grateful indeed that he had given me this golden opportunity to return to practice. I determined there and then that when the time was right, if circumstances allowed, I would continue my career. Meanwhile I did and saw as much as possible, shuddering at the memory of my confidence as a student and at the narrow escapes my patients had so often had.

My husband, whose interest and work lay in the field of industrial engineering, was working as a consultant at that time, giving his expert knowledge of new methods for the improvement of labour, for increased work output, for streamlining, to every factory that solicited his services. Before the children were much older we left the Eastern Cape and undertook the marathon move to the Eastern Transvaal by motor-car, a distance of about 1,200 miles. With us travelled our exuberant young boxer, who loved every moment of the trip, and an under-tranquillised kitten which needed a booster quarter-grain of Luminal every four hours throughout the entire journey.

My husband's family owned a magnificent estate in the Lowveld district of the Eastern Transvaal, mainly citrus and subtropical crops but also, like the whole area, well-endowed with stock of all types. Because of the local need for a veterinarian (there wasn't a private vet for hundreds of miles each way at that time), and since my husband encouraged me to continue my work, and provided me with excellent facilities, I found myself in the full swing of general practice within six months.

The children and I did not remain in the valley for more than a year. At that time my marriage was heading for disaster, and we mutually decided to call it a day and part ways. After the divorce we moved to the little village of White River, only fifteen miles away, a charming centre of the farming community about 1,000 ft. higher in the hills. Although the population there is very small, it took only a day or two before the word got around that there was a new vet in the district. People trooped in with flowers, cakes and good wishes, examining everything from my microscope and shiny instruments on the shelves to my professional plate, nailed up outside the door: 'Veterinary Surgeon, *Dierearts*'. If only my Professor of Surgery could see me now! All I needed was my first patient, and finally he came too – a donkey with a sore foot, and we led him right into the second room to the vast enjoyment of the watching crowd.

I must have seemed optimistic. No vet had ever succeeded in White River: it simply did not pay. And yet farmers were becoming gradually more vet-conscious, and competitions at local shows increased in the livestock sections. On the face of it, it seemed foolhardy, especially for a woman, to go into mixed practice; on the other hand, I had the advantage that since I *was* a woman, people wanted to see if I could do the job. There was no other private vet in the area in those days; farmers had no choice but to call me.

That first day we were drinking coffee out of any receptacle we could find – crucibles, beakers – using glass rods to stir the sugar. I possessed three cups and two saucers at the time, but the coffee seemed to taste better somehow when drunk in an unconventional manner. Sometimes the taste was slightly unusual, or even the colour, but hardly anyone noticed these bizarre effects.

A young man burst into the crowded room; he was tall and handsome, but very flustered. "I say, are you by any chance the new vet?" he said in a cultured English voice which quite belied his unkempt dress. His shirt was hanging out, and through it a hairy suntanned chest was exposed: the one and only button that was done up was anchored by a long and flimsy thread. His trousers were torn and his *veldskoene* (rough boots used much for comfortable working wear) added to the effect, covering his large feet in a haphazard sort of manner. He peered at me, a little surprised, but whatever his thoughts, he kept them wisely to himself. "Have some coffee," I invited, upon which he gratefully sank upon the little stool, took off his misty glasses and wiped the perspiration from his eyes and face. "I say, it is a hot day! Coffee will be just the thing." I hesitated to ask what I could do for him: perhaps he had only come to take a look at me; on the other hand – and my heart sang with joy at the prospect – perhaps he was a potential client with a problem. Coffee was of the instant variety, the boiling water being added directly from the steriliser. (Months later, this same young man was enjoying some eleven o'clock refreshment with me, when I noticed that he turned a pale greenish colour, and hastily put down his cup. "Anything wrong?" I asked. "I say, what have you been boiling up in your steriliser? There is some ghastly thing or other floating about on top of the coffee!" I looked, and sure enough there it was, a certain unmentionable object derived from an operation that I had just performed on a cat. Poor Michael; he took it all rather more seriously than I would have expected, but then a man would perhaps take it that way. Henceforth I brought a flask of boiling water from the house, and on this understanding my friend continued to drop in for his eleven o'clock refreshment.)

The young man suddenly leaped to his feet, tucked his shirt into his sagging trousers, declared that he felt infinitely better, and would I now come with him at once, to see his cow, which was about to burst; her udder had already reached an enormous size when he left the farm. I was taken completely by surprise, but acting on reflex, I took up my medical bag, grabbed an overall, called my African orderly, and leapt into the station-wagon. I followed my client for about twelve miles until at last we reached his farm. The cow in question was in the driveway, an enormous Friesland, with the most wonderful udder and teats imaginable. An African was hosing her down, while she stood placidly chewing the cud. I almost wept with relief, for on the journey I had visualised the most terrifying possibilities and was not at all sure whether I would be able to cope with any of them. "You are a lucky man," I said, "your cow has the most beautiful udder I have ever seen. When she calves, you will have enough milk to supply the whole of the village! Why were you worried about her?" The distracted young man then revealed that he had never owned a cow before, and had just acquired this one; he knew less than nothing about udders, calving and general bovine care. He acted exactly like an expectant father, and I could visualise him pacing the cow-stall in the same manner as expectant fathers are supposed to do when waiting for their first baby to emerge. I attempted to reassure him, promising to come at a moment's notice if there was any difficulty at all. In actual fact this magnificent cow calved while he was asleep that same night and has born many calves since, rewarding his anxiety by never giving him less than seven gallons of the most delicious milk.

Within a few months the practice became very busy and I began to do my long-distance calls at crack of dawn, sometimes leaving even before dawn. In this way I could do a full day's work by two o'clock, when the children came out of school. After that I only attended the emergencies, spending my time at home or taking the children with me on my rounds. The most vivid dawn episode came early on in my veterinary life, in midsummer, just one month after my consulting-rooms were opened. I particularly wished to reach my client before the sun was up, for the task that lay ahead was a *post mortem* on a cow already dead two days, that sort of work being best carried out before breakfast and before the heat of the day.

I drove thirty miles to reach the homestead and knocked loudly on the door of a very silent house, finding the complete lack of activity rather disconcerting. I was just wondering if, after all, I had reached the wrong homestead (having little bump of locality, I had become used to losing my way) when the door was opened, and I saw a half-clad form squinting at me through the dim sunrise light, with an expression of one who has just woken from a nightmare and who has not yet shaken it off.

I did not catch his first sentence completely, but gathered that it indicated a question as to whether I had lost my way or my mind or both. I explained meekly who I was, trying instinctively not to raise my voice too much, for I have heard it said that sleepwalkers should be awakened gently, if at all. I patiently pointed out the reasons for my early intrusion which sounded good enough to me, but seemed to arouse some doubt in the mind of my client. Having (as I thought) convinced him that my presence was not only decent but necessary, I suggested, more emphatically this time, that since I had come this long way to catch the early morning coolness, we would be well advised to start at once. Upon this, the farmer seemed suddenly to come to life, and as though for protection against an immoral suggestion, loudly called for his son, who had obviously not missed a single word of our conversation, judging from the sheepish expression on his face. "But we expected a man *veearts* (vet)," said the father belligerently, "the chemist didn't say you is a woman!" He then proceeded to examine me minutely as though to convince himself of my sex, taking me in from my long hair to my feet, till I felt very embarrassed. In those early days of practice I had not yet achieved a definite technique for dealing with such cases, and only later acquired a successful counter-method to such tactics of intimidation.

"*Ek is jammer* (I am sorry)," I said, "that you have gained the wrong impression. However, I was created this way, and now let us get on with the job." We filed up the hill, the father still grumbling under his breath about the emancipation of woman: I was armed with a rubber apron, two very long knives high in my black boots, and my African orderly followed.

The body of the cow lay half a mile away; by this time the morning light was accentuating the gross distension of the beast. The first incision in a case like this usually brings a strong gust of unpleasantness, so I advised my client to stand well back to avoid it. He proudly stuck out his chin at the suggestion, stood firm and gave the impression that I had offended him deeply by implying that I could survive such an ordeal better than he. While absorbed in my gruesome work I happened to glance up just in time to see the farmer staggering drunkenly away, hand to mouth, his face a sickly green.

Half an hour later we assembled round the kitchen table to drink strong home-brewed coffee and 'dunk' (dip) our rusks, as is the custom. I had been able to reached the definite diagnosis of Blackquarter, explaining the course of this dreaded disease as fully as possible. I stopped speaking and an uneasy silence followed, while all eyes turned towards the elder of the house, now restored to normal composure. "Well, I am jiggered," he finally exploded, "*ek is vragtig verbaas* (I am really amazed); you work like a man without even changing colour. How do you manage to do such work, and still look like a woman?" Coming from him, I took this as a compliment and was just beginning to erase his previous antagonism from my memory, when he continued: "Why don't you behave normal like other women, stay at the house and have children and get a good man to cook for, instead of messing around in cows' insides? You listen to me, my *meisie* (girl), and change before it's too late."

With these words I departed and drove to my next call with his warning ringing in my ears, kicking myself mentally for not having explained that one *can* work and cook and have children all at the same time; or can one? Had I told him the story of my life, he would doubtlessly not have believed me, and small wonder, for I myself often find the circumstances of my existence a surprise. In the course of time I grew to love these farmers, tough, straightforward, very generous and honest. What an effort it must have cost them to suppress their antiquated cavemen views on the role of woman in society, and to continue to seek my advice and my services.

The next call took me into the lovely Heidelberg valley. This range of hills, though it lies adjacent to the White River area, seems very different from the surrounding country both in atmosphere and vegetation. Leaving the main tar road, we turned west and in a few moments had entered a different world. Originally one man had owned all these lands, and gradually they were cut up and sold; the divisions were made with infinite care, the farmers were imbued with a pioneering, hard-working spirit. The soil is very fertile here; although there is a large amount of rock, this has been skilfully used in the creation of gardens. There is no shortage of water, and the contrast of stone and brilliantly coloured shrubs and flowers on different levels is very picturesque. Due to a kind climate and local artistry, there is a continuance of colour all through the year. Autumn changes are not greatly in evidence, though spring brings bursts of new leaf and blossoms, a reminder that in this northern part of southern Africa, Nature has not lost her awareness of the changing seasons.

I was to visit the main Rottcher farmstead; this would be a very long call for I had come to take blood from each of eighty wild cattle, to test them for Contagious Abortion, which had caused heavy calf losses and which was threatening human health through contaminated milk. I had often worked here before and in spite of the task ahead looked forward to it; on this farm I was always treated rather like a china doll, by both the farm-manager and the African workers, a pleasant change from the usual attitude of being regarded as sexless and invulnerable.

I knew everything would be ready for me on arrival; this was also exceptional, for almost everywhere the vet is kept waiting, the excuse being that he is always late in any case. There would be quite a lot of excitement on a morning like this. On other farms I usually joined in the rodeo which controlling wild bovines naturally entails. The herd was restrained by driving them, twenty at a time, into a crush where they were packed like sardines to prevent movement. One by one the animals were brought forward and dealt with, each one trussed up and tied, the horns steadied and secured, the nose held by means of a 'bull noseholder'. It made quite a scene; amidst the choking dust which the heaving, rebellious beasts kicked up, to the rhythmical incantations which the Zulu labourers use to calm the beasts, I had to find my way, place a *riem* (thong made of cow hide) round the neck of each beast to bring up the jugular vein and then plunge a needle into it. There was usually some additional struggle and disturbance at the first prick, but after that, providing the animal could be held, the collection of the blood into the small bleeding-bottles provided was a simple matter.

In spite of the excellent restraint it happened quite often that some specially powerful cow would break the human barrier. Animals hate to be interrupted in their daily routine, and regard such interference with great apprehension and suspicion. On this occasion the young manager came off lightly and only sustained some grazes when he was dragged forward by a wild-eyed Afrikander cow who was determined to return to her calf. Holding on to her lance-like horns, the manager managed at last to slow her down and in spite of loud bellows the fugitive was once more held fast and subdued. This incident did much to boost the manager's morale, for everyone knows that it takes enormous strength and much courage to check a full-grown Afrikander cow, bent on returning to her calf.

I finally left the farm at eleven o'clock, very pleased to have the eighty bottles of blood safely stowed on the back seat of the station-wagon, to be sent to the Veterinary Research station that day, after the marking and cleaning process was completed. On the way back to my consulting-rooms, my Zulu orderly and I shared some sandwiches, thoughtfully and lovingly packed by my maid, who has never tired of insisting that I am underfed and overworked. I suspect that she has a target in mind which is closely connected with her own Herculean measurements. Little does she know that if I ever reached such earthshaking circumference I would not only lose my entire male clientele, but also the agility which every country vet must possess, and without which he would become a very bad risk for Medical Insurance.

Had it been earlier I would have stopped somewhere along the way, as is my habit at breakfast-time, and burst unceremoniously into some friendly household in time to join this most enjoyable repast of the day. In the Lowveld the 'breakfast habit' has become fairly general practice. In the hot summer months, when hours of work have already been done by eight o'clock, it is a wonderful break to spend some time relaxing over the breakfast table, seeing one's friends while the air is still deliciously cool and fresh.

My surgery is placed in a side-street of the village between the barber and the butcher, both patient silent sufferers of the sounds and smells which daily emanate from my doors and windows. Across the road is a native store which incessantly plays the latest Bantu hit music; having very little alternative, I decided to become interested in this form of rhythmic sound, rather than resist it and head towards a term in a strait-jacket. Next door to the barber are the rooms of the doctor, a general practitioner, who usually has a large African clientele queueing at the back and past my windows. The cry of a baby and that of a Siamese cat are very alike; the doctor's nurse has on occasion dropped everything and come running in to placate what she thought to be a baby in pain, only to find an indignant Siamese Temple cat vocalising upon the table.

My barber neighbour not only puts up smilingly with the howls and barks which stream forth, but actually seems to enjoy the excitement; he has told me that he would miss me terribly were I ever to move. He efficiently sharpens my post-mortem knives and scissors on his barber's strap, and sometimes stores animals to await my coming when the surgery is closed. His own clients suffer the impositions that I put upon him, thus proving beyond doubt that he must be a pastmaster of his art, and that people will endure anything to get the best.

There came a time, however, when even my saintly neighbour made objection: I had a sheep carcase on my surgery table, and instead of insisting that it be put back on to the truck and there dissecting it, I proceeded to open it on the spot. The result was disastrous. An old gentleman was having a haircut at that exact moment, and almost succumbed to the terrible fumes; the waiting clients filed out of the shop in silent horror for this was too high a price to pay even for an expert haircut. The barber, for the first time, ventured to complain in a most restrained and polite manner; putting only his head round the door (a very courageous action, under the circumstances) he looked at me with doleful eyes while his kind face turned ashen-grey at what he witnessed on the table. As he slid away as silently as he had come, I had the strong impression that if anyone could be assured of a place in heaven, it would surely be he.

As I pulled up outside the surgery I was met by a most welcome and familiar sight: the silver-grey caravan of my unconventional friends, the Sinclairs. It was unusual to see them in the Lowveld at this time of year, for it was the perfect winter climate which usually brought them back to us. The two Sinclairs, complete with two children, Land-Rover and caravan-truck are an Australian couple who have travelled far and wide, living a nomad life for the past ten years. Bill is a professional photographer of high standing in the field of wild life, but perhaps his talent for storytelling and his vocabulary of swear-words are equally great.

His wife, a sylph-like girl, has a forceful personality which matches her husband's and assists him wonderfully in his work. She seems to have the worst of the bargain, for not only does she give her two boys tuition by correspondence course, but it is she, alone, who co-ordinates the mobile home, cooks the meals, develops the negatives in their convertible kitchen, and collects the hard-earned money – which is then immediately spent on some item of photographic equipment. Then Bill goes off to get bread-and-butter commissions – child studies, which he hates, and photographs of people's homes – so that their day-to-day living costs can be met.

This foursome was something of a curiosity; Bill had piloted aeroplanes during the war, had sailed a yacht round the world, and had done many other interesting things, and he knew how to spin a yarn about his adventures. They made life-long friends and bitter enemies, mainly the latter; they quarrelled with enjoyment, but never with each other; they took offence in the flash of an eye. Their decisions were made almost entirely on the spur of the moment; when they looked most settled, drinking tea peacefully in my house, a not-a-care-in-the-world expression on their faces, they would suddenly leap up, bundle their belongings into the caravan, and off they would go, declaring that they were tired of the Lowveld and the bums who lived in it. But they would be sure to come back sooner or later. They would then travel on to wherever their fancy took them – truly free as most people would like to be, yet standing up remarkably well to the trial of living on top of each other day after day.

Criticism followed them wherever they went, and they received it with equanimity or with extreme rudeness; their reactions were unpredictable, I believe, even to themselves. Nan was the most aggressive partner, able to spit from behind her waist-long gipsy-like mane like an enraged leopardess. When they made an appearance there was bound to be something new, something different. I was always delighted to have them around.

Before I had time to reach the door, they were upon me, "Hi, kid!" said Bill. He gave me a fatherly pat on my back, and burst into that wonderful ear to ear smile of his which always made me feel much better. "Same old Sue, haven't changed at all," he muttered happily and to my intense satisfaction. He always greeted me this way, whatever time interval had elapsed; I was greatly relieved, for the day might well come when he would say, "Hi, kid, growing a bit long in the tooth!" The children came running out; Spike, rather small for his six years, with his cherub face and ever-dripping nose; Butch, his thirteen-year-old brother, uncannily like his father in voice and manner and looks. He was always spoiling for a good fight and would stand up for his brother against anything and anyone when the need arose.

The surgery was full of animal and human life and there I found Nan, drinking tea with my long-suffering secretary. She was the only one who welcomed me; my secretary's patience was ebbing fast, for she was trying to keep people and animals at bay at the same time, a truly formidable task. I was an hour late for my appointments and badly in need of a wash, so I gave them a placatory smile, and asked what was in the big basket on the desk. Whatever it was, it seemed to have an unnerving effect on the patients. I was momentarily stunned when they told me that there were twenty-four mice inside, waiting to be sexed. "Food for the python," Nan said almost pityingly, as though only a fool like me could ask such a lunatic question. "Not pets, I assure you. Must keep the females; the python eats the males, one a day."

I saw my clients visibly shudder and draw away from my unusual friend. No one asked where the python was: this stranger-than-fiction amazon might well have her pet curled up inside her shirt. I went into the next room to wash and change, and I must have considerably startled the waiting-room with a loud howl not unlike that of one of my Siamese patients, which I could not repress. The python was in the wash-basin, obviously enjoying herself immensely. "Don't worry about her," Nan said nonchalantly, "I just put her in there for her bath. She has to have it once a day before her meal."

The lady with the bird-cage, waiting to have her budgie's beak cut, got up, protectingly clasping the cage as close to her as she could, mumbled something about coming back another day, and went out. The other clients bravely stayed on while Nan extricated her snake from the basin and placed it in an empty basket. Everyone was extremely interested as Nan took a mouse from the other basket, asked me to sex it, and when reassured that it was a male, killed it and held it out for the python. The latter eyed it speculatively for a few moments, gripped it in its jaws and slowly and gradually swallowed it, while we watched the process with absolute fascination. "She is particularly temperamental after she has fed," Nan said. "It is the only time when she is aggressive towards us. Just put your hand on her and see." I placed my hand on the cold, muscular, rippling body and immediately she reared up, hissing rather like a miniature dragon. "Lucky that she is still a baby," I said. "It reminds me of the only wild python I have ever seen at close quarters, on the way to the Gorongosa Game Sanctuary." Memories came flooding back, and the sound and smells and textures of that experience.

CHAPTER 4

Of Lions, Elephants and Pythons

My children and I had developed an interested awareness of wild life, encouraged in this by many friends who had lived in the Lowveld all their lives, and whose knowledge of the subject was therefore tremendous. For me it was a completely new world; I found myself growing up all over again with my children – I had never, in my own childhood, been able to live as I chose. They had all the things I had dreamed of: pigeons, dogs, cats, guinea-pigs, donkeys, horses, cows, and behind all this a spacious environment: I enjoyed it doubly, relishing their childhood freedom with them. I had grown up in countries where lions walked unhappily in cramped cages, where the bizarre shapes and sizes of zoo animals seemed remote and irrelevant.

News was drifting down from a newly opened Game Sanctuary in northern Mozambique, eleven hundred miles away, said to be yet unspoilt and filled with game. A group of us decided to go and investigate 'Gorongosa', so named after the province in which it lies; we chose June as a suitable month, for at that time the heat is still bearable and the waters have usually receded after the big rains.

We left in two vehicles: Eddie and Ann Haig, a farmer friend with his wife, Christopher and Roger Pike, two young bachelor brothers, another farmer-photographer named Howard Kirk and myself. The journey took us first through the northern Transvaal and across the mountain passes to Rhodesia; we stopped at Umtali for repairs, and took the opportunity of taking a look at this lovely mountain-ringed town, a hundred and sixty miles west of our destination.

Soon we were travelling towards the frontier post at some considerable speed, and I was soundly asleep on the back seat of the station-wagon. Suddenly there was a terrible screeching of brakes; we came to a halt, and I was thrown from my comfortable resting-place with an abrupt jerk. Before I could collect my wits, Howard and Christopher had leaped out, and a moment later I was rubbing my eyes in disbelief to see them gripping each one end of a python which stretched the full width of the road. Jumping out in alarm, I asked them what on earth they thought they were doing. I should have guessed that it was all in a good cause; Howard has a touching tenderness for all God's creatures, and would rather suffer injury himself than allow harm to come to any animal or bird or insect.

"I am afraid we may have injured it," he said with his usual calm. "Please examine it minutely before we let it go. It would be better to destroy it, if it is going to suffer." As I obediently palpated its body piece by piece, I was tremendously impressed by the crushing power within the rippling body, thick as a man's arm. A giant compared to the baby python I found in the surgery wash basin almost a year later.

"Let go, and get out of the way." We leapt aside but Howard, watching for our safety, was the last to release the uninjured snake which struck viciously at his knee, then slid at lightning speed across the road and into long grass. Its disappearance was so quick that for a moment I wondered if it could really have been there a moment ago. I examined Howard's knee and was allowed to paint it with disinfectant, while our hero grumbled at the unnecessary loss of time. We knew that such a bite was not venomous, and yet an infection could easily set in: fangs of a reptile are like the teeth of a cat, and the resultant wounds almost always turn septic. In fact the bite turned out to be so deep that he bears a scar to this day as a memento of that episode.

Having crossed the border-post in the afternoon, we reached Villa Machados at dusk, hoping that we might still be able to cross the Pungwe river into the Sanctuary that night, and settle into camp before the next day. We stopped at a small local inn to make inquiries, but found that the landlord, a jovial rotund Portuguese, had other ideas. He assured us that we would have to find accommodation there with him that night, since any unwary traveller who entered the Park after dark would probably never be seen again. In his very amusing, broken lingo, he gave us a graphic description of how this disappearance would be brought about. "The elfant just go fipps and dat de end." These words were accompanied by a suitable gesture, our host making a wide

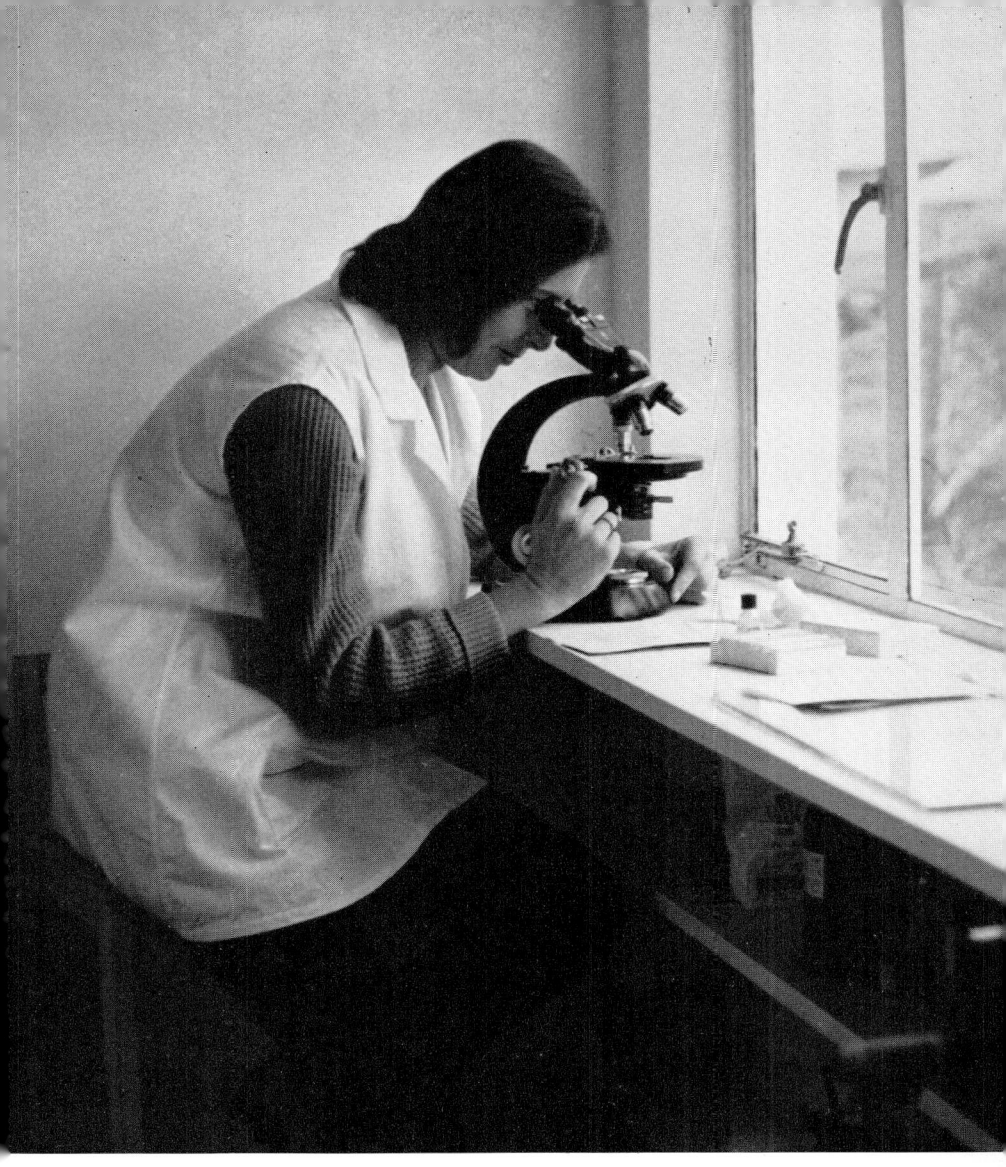

1. The author and her microscope.

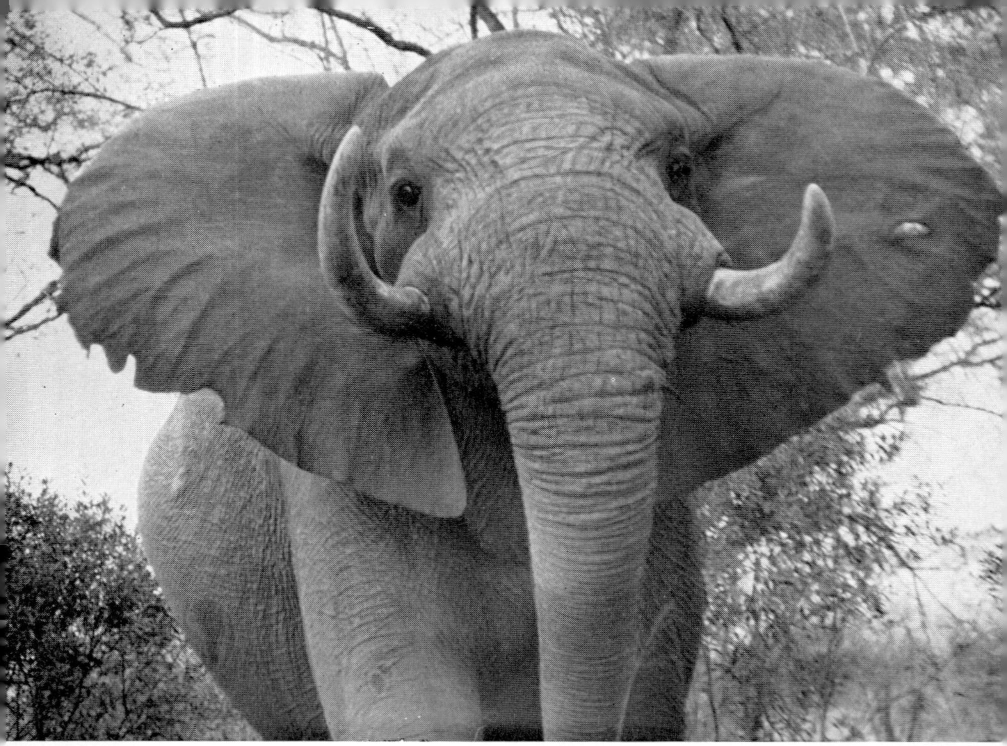

2. Herd sentry.

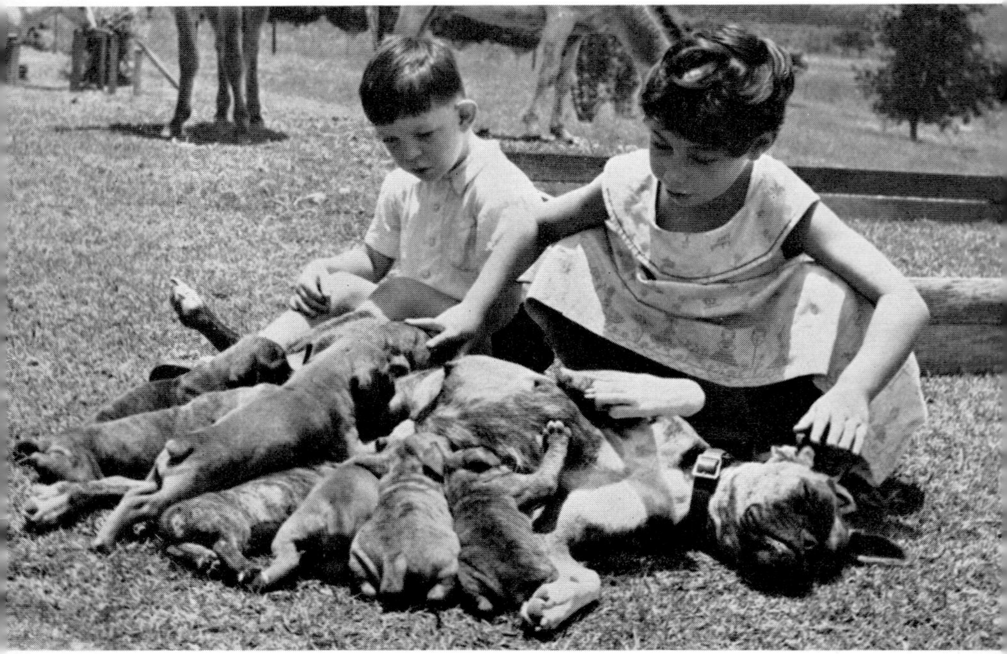

3. The author's children, Guy and Gail, when very young with some of their pets.

OF LIONS, ELEPHANTS AND PYTHONS

circling movement with his arm, no doubt to represent the elephant's trunk, and accompanying this by a threatening, almost elephantine grimace, making his meaning all too clear. "Zo, he take you." There was such finality in his words that we felt forced to believe him, and decided to make the best of the evening by drowning our disappointment in the heady Portuguese wine.

We wondered afterwards if the risk involved in staying at this unspeakably unhygienic inn had not been greater than any possible danger from elephants. The accommodation was most inadequate; we could distinguish about four different varieties of cockroaches, and had an uncomfortable feeling that the place was crawling with all sorts of other and more unspeakable horrors. Had it not been for Ann Haig's foresight in bringing a Flit bomb along, we would have spent an entirely sleepless night; as it was, the previous night's repast (consisting mainly of the flesh of a very old buffalo, fried in green oil of unknown origin) played havoc with our digestions. We left before dawn, eager to leave this little nightmare behind, hoping to be on the ferry and well away with the first light.

Crossing the river at dawn was an unforgettable experience; the water was calm and blue, the banks of the river thick with vivid tropical shrubs and trees. Life was beginning to stir in the upmost branches; we seemed to have disturbed some vervet monkeys, for we could hear them chattering in the most animated monkey-fashion, clearly discussing us in great detail. The ferryman made a swift and smooth landing, touching Gorongosa soil at last; and then from the banks of the river we continued without a stop, hoping to make up some of the time we had lost.

Driving through dense jungle along a well-kept sand road we frequently stopped to admire eland, most royal and lovely of the larger antelope, which do not abound in our bushveld areas. At eight o'clock, just as we were developing a ravenous appetite, we came upon a breeding herd of elephants blocking the road. Our friends on the other side of the river had warned us several times to keep our engines running at all costs when such a herd was close, for elephants in these parts are still unused to man and motor, and will charge at the slightest provocation, especially when young are at foot. We enjoyed the sight for over half an hour before the cows and their brood began to move off into the forest; gradually the herd followed and let us pass. We drank in this magnificent scene, especially the little ones tugging thirstily from their mothers, straining just behind the front legs, not quite knowing which way to curl their trunks. They had been aware of us all the time, and once the watchman of the herd had thrown up his trunk and trumpeted a warning which rang and echoed through the forest like a fanfare. Since we did not move but remained quietly in our vehicles, he had calmed down and the young had resumed their repast.

The day had warmed up considerably by the time we reached camp; we settled in at Chitiengo, showered and took our bearings. One is unfortunately not permitted to camp or cook one's own meals here; one has to make use of the main restaurant. Thus everything becomes centralised; Mozambique Africans – blacker than the Zulus or the Swazis, of taller stature with oval-shaped heads – make the most amusing companions and knowledgeable guides, and one is not permitted to go out without one of them. Without knowing any of the native tongues and without any knowledge of English on their part, we somehow knew exactly where we were going and why. Eddie Haig had built a hardwood screen to fit in to the back of his open truck and this enabled us to travel together standing on the back, taking photographs through the peep holes in this mobile hide.

That morning we set forth, full of anticipation, prepared for anything. The floods had only just receded the month before, and so the water-drenched land was beautifully lush. The great plains of green were teeming with game. In our wildest dreams we had never imagined such herds of water-buck, zebra, buffalo and wildebeest. We gazed across to the distant mountains, still within the Reserve, but inaccessible at this time of year. There were groups of elephants in every direction, three thousand altogether at the latest count within an area of two thousand square miles.

We were guided to an old disused camp near the Urema river, which forms the northern boundary of the Park. A few years ago the floods had completely swamped the site and since that time the lions had claimed it as their own domain. They were certainly in possession that morning. We could see them sprawled everywhere; on the roof of one cottage lay a huge, black-maned lion, who must have climbed the stone steps to reach the sun-roof top.

They lay on the cool stone floors of the cottages, glaring at us out of the doorways rather as one might regard a group of unwelcome intruders.

I did not feel very secure in the open truck, with no protection but that boarding screen; frequently one lion or another would charge with some spirit – though our guide saw it as mere bravado, as his contemptuous gestures indicated. For the photographers this was sheer heaven; they remained glued to their cameras for over an hour, while I listened apprehensively to the fierce growling resentment of the lions at our intrusion. Only the previous day we had watched a lioness dragging a freshly killed wildebeest into the shade of a palm tree; I was acutely conscious of the immense strength that those jaws possess.

Eventually, and to my intense relief, we moved on to the Urema river, stopping about a quarter of a mile from the water's edge since our guide, Tickey, pointed out that we would get stuck if we drove farther. We walked on and a gruesome sight met our eyes: a partially devoured hippopotamus protruded from the water while myriads of crocodiles feasted on the distended carcase. We were told that for two days two bull hippos had battled along this stretch of the immense river, causing a tremendous uproar, until at last one had been vanquished.

The next day, not very far from this horrific scene, we saw a herd of hippos peacefully immersed in the shallows at the edge of the huge river, and among them a rose-coloured – yes, a *pink* hippo – baby! Wondering at first if this was the effect of the wine-party the night before, and deciding that if this was the case all the hippos would be pink, we came to the conclusion that it must be an albino – a very rare thing indeed. Our friends would never believe us, we thought, and correctly: when told of this strange apparition, they refused to accept the idea at all, putting it down to the hot climate and the cumulative effect of fermented grape juice. The only proof we had was a colour slide, but this did not accurately record the rosiness of the young hippo, which, lying close to its mother, merged with the colour of its mother's skin and the watery environment.

Next morning, we made the acquaintance of the Warden, Senhor Roderigues; he invited us to go with him and honoured us by climbing on to the back of the truck, which commanded an excellent view. This warm-hearted Portuguese, who was once an army officer, regarded the Game Reserve as his 'farm', and tenderly protected and watched over his animals with immense pride and devotion.

Panting in the shade of a huge fig-tree lay a single lion, an unusual sight at that time of year, which was the mating season: Senhor Rodrigues greeted him as Chico, the tailless one, and told us that he was known to be of a much fiercer disposition than the others. Even the natives, he explained, are terrified of this beast, which charges at the slightest provocation. Perhaps he had developed an inferiority complex due to his tailless condition.

We left the truck and were led to the private pool of an old, cast-out hippo bull known as Joâo. At first we could not see him, for the pool was covered in cabbage-like water plants through which not an inch of water was visible. Rodrigues threw a pebble on to the surface, and at once a huge hippo head emerged, draped in vegetation. We managed to get some good photos of this incredible and amusing hermit, particularly of his immense jaws and mouth which he opened as fully as he could, giving us an unforgettable view of his tonsils.

We discovered that the Game Reserve has an immense variety of vegetation, for the plains had, at this point, melted into grassy expanses scattered with palm-trees and not as open as the wide plains. Thickets of palms formed excellent cover for the lions. Cruising along at an easy speed, we came upon a group feeding on the remains of a wildebeest. Dangerously close at hand, we found eland, grazing in company with zebra and impala; they doubtlessly felt safe since the hunters' appetite was temporarily assuaged. There were nine in this pride, the cubs behaving exactly as other infants would at the end of a feast; they were making battle over the last of the juicy bones, tugging and growling to gain possession. Their elders, ignoring them completely, rose one by one to drink from the near-by river, which gave the appearance of a solid and serpentine band of yellow and orange water-plants. Above, the vultures cruised in and out of the palm-trees, causing a continuous rustling of the dry leaves as they alighted and almost immediately launched again into flight. At last, unable to contain their hungry impatience any longer, they landed among the lions and began to tear at pieces of entrails which they had discarded. At the far side four young males were lying cheek by jowl, licking the last drops of wildebeest blood off each other's cheeks.

On the way back to the camp we were thrilled by the sight of a large herd of buffalo in motion. Having unwittingly caused a stampede, we sat spellbound, listening to the pounding hoofs and watching the solid mass gradually disappear over the horizon. Coming across a small group later, we approached carefully and hardly disturbed two old-timers; they were surrounded by egrets, the so-called tick-birds, which contrasted in their pure white to the thick mud-caked brown-black of the buffalo hides. These patriarchs were very little discomfited by our presence. One of them, complete with ox-pecker upon his back, stared unwinkingly at us while continuing to chew the cud. From side to side in rotary motion went his jaws, the peaceful rhythm giving the lie to his fierce temperament; it is said that the buffalo is the most dangerous of all the hunter's adversaries, and the most wily. Near Chitiengo, we met Tusco, the single-tusked elephant bull; Warden Rodrigues described him as a lovable but somewhat unpredictable character, for he was lonely and old, and perhaps, like Chico, he suffered from a psychological kink, due to the imperfection of his appearance.

It had been a wonderful and very full day; we cooled off under the showers, for the temperature had risen over 80 degrees. The iced *cerveige*, a delicious Portuguese beer, was a real life-saver at this end of the day, and we imbibed until it was dark and time for dinner. A young Portuguese joined us at our long table, bringing his guitar with him and giving a melodious finishing touch to the full and glorious day.

Just before we were due to leave I was asked to sort out an unusual problem, one that most vets would relish. The Warden had come upon the body of a cow elephant early that morning, attended by two grief-stricken calves. These two had immediately charged him, and he had been forced to seek refuge in the nearest tree. Much later, when their resentment had abated, they abandoned the body but hovered in that part of the forest for some days. They would probably be adopted by an 'auntie' elephant in the near future, and thus have protection and guidance until they reached maturity.

The warden now asked me to perform a post-mortem on the

carcase to establish the cause of death. I readily agreed to the attempt, though I was unfamiliar with elephantine anatomy, and had no idea where to begin. When we arrived at the scene it was already a hive of activity, for the Africans had opened the body and carefully disembowelled it, laying the different organs on the ground in the most haphazard fashion; thus my problem of where to begin was made even more difficult.

I spent some time examining the various regions and organs, after a preliminary period of trying to orientate myself; the large dimensions, the uncertain identity of what I examined caused me considerable confusion. To me, all this was a professional delight; but to my long-suffering patient friends, it meant a morning spent among the ghastly mess of entrails, buzzing with flies, as the sun became a vertical shaft of heat. At last I established the cause of death: it was a case of peritonitis of the large (very large) bowel, possibly caused by a tusk injury, and one which must have been inflicted some time ago. The lesions were not fresh, and the elephant must have died of septicaemia after a period of intense pain and suffering.

It suddenly occurred to me to search for the uterus; I had visions of returning to White River with yet another embryo to add to my collection, this one pickled in the best Portuguese white wine. Having failed to find anything resembling a uterus, I entered the enormous body of the elephant, knife in hand, and more or less disappeared inside to search further. After some time I discovered, to my great disappointment, that there was no foetus present; I was glad, however, to re-enter the world of light and space. The Warden and Africans were staring at me with consternation, for by this time I was caked in elephant blood, and the accompanying odour was strongly offensive. The Warden muttered something which, I thought, resembled the words 'very unladylike', but I was probably wrong, and his muttering would probably have been in Portuguese, anyway. He thanked me profusely for solving the mystery, promising me the tail of the elephant as a memento of the occasion, which promise he kept. As we drove off the Africans were already cutting the meat with great dexterity preparing for the feast which was to follow that night.

My friends begged me to restore myself to my normal colour and odour as quickly as possible, for the sweet stench that emanated was almost unbearable. I reappeared after an hour, none the worse for wear, although I felt as if the topmost layer of skin had been removed in the violent process of scrubbing. In spite of my intense ablutions, for some days following, whenever I was downwind, one of our party would curl up his nose and dryly remark that he could smell elephant blood.

That night we slept, or attempted to sleep, to the ghoulish chorus of many hyenas; they were anticipating their share of the meat which was drying in strips in front of huge fires at the edge of the camp. This was not an unusual procedure, but to us it brought visions of cannibal days, and we realised the intensity of the African's need and love for meat. They had erected temporary drying racks which faced the fires and not daring to leave their spoil for a moment, they had curled up on the spot, protecting their precious fare from the ravenous carrion-eaters. In spite of these precautions, the hyenas managed to steal some of the meat during the night: leaving plenty, however, for the indignant natives. For a European-bred person, like myself, this scene held absolute fascination: this was Africa in the raw, the primitive interplay between man and the wild.

Some days later, Howard, anxious to get all the photographs of lions that he could, asked me to drive him in the very early morning so that we could be undisturbed. Very soon – at Gorongosa one seldom goes far without spotting game – we saw lions across the plain, and were able to approach slowly to within a range of ten to fifteen yards. A magnificently maned male lay in apparently deep sleep next to his mate; but his sleep was shallow and he was up in a flash, yawning and stretching one moment, charging us the next. He had probably been disturbed by some movement inside our station wagon, and he came at us with real anger, stopping short only at the uncomfortable distance of about five feet. At this point he admitted his bluff and retreated back into sleep.

We watched their peaceful twitchings for about ten minutes, when suddenly the lion rose and the mating prelude began. This lasted for two or three minutes, the lioness remaining recumbent on her chest throughout. After mating, as the roaring and moaning of the pair subsided, the lion detached himself, and within moments they were again a picture of complete relaxation. During the hour we spent watching this spectacle, the pair mated four times at regular intervals. On the fourth occasion the lioness, in a testy mood, repulsed the male with angry snarls. The lion, as though looking for sympathy, retreated and approached us in leisurely fashion, ambling up to the window, and fixing us through it with an amber-eyed stare. At this point my self-protective reflex asserted itself and I drove off, relieved to see him standing in our wake. I learnt afterwards that mating is repeated over about a week or so, during which time lions do not hunt at all, but spend their days in pairs, very touchy and aggressive when disturbed.

The day arrived when we had to leave this idyllic country, but even in a week we had seen and heard and learnt enough to keep us thinking for a lifetime. Before returning to the ferry we drove to the water pans adjoining the open plains, said to be an assembly-place for myriads of birds. This was certainly no exaggeration. Here different species of herons, rare elsewhere, lived in great numbers; the Goliath, white and purple herons mixed with the saddle-bill stork and the carnivorous maribu, the latter feeding on a carcase alongside a group of vultures. There were sea-gulls and pelicans, plovers and coursers, living and feeding side by side. The sea-eagle appeared, sending his haunting call across the vast expanses. Many varieties of rollers, eagles, doves, ibis, hornbills, ducks and geese have made this their home. A crocodile, stretched on the bank of a pool, lay immobile as a statue, his upper jaw wide open while the blacksmith plover apparently cleaned his teeth. We must have disturbed this prehistoric shape on the bank, for suddenly his huge jaws shut and he slithered into the water, an amazing contrast to the bird-song and the beating of many-coloured wings.

On the way out we stopped for a few moments among the yellow-stemmed fever-trees; they stand strangely aloof in their great height and only unbend to the elephant when he chooses to reach up with his great trunk and bring their branches crashing down. The trees in this part of Africa are too high even for giraffe, and for this reason there is not a single giraffe to be found here.

It is interesting that in the East African Rift Valley the giraffe have adapted themselves to feeding from the small acacia trees, bending downwards while they eat. One wonders whether here in Gorongosa, the giraffe has disappeared because of an inadequate or ill-placed food supply.

Near-by, a very big elephant was dusting himself; we watched him through our binoculars, and saw that one of his hind legs was caught in a snare, and that it was oozing and raw. He supported his weight on three legs, his injured limb only just touching the ground. It was an ugly sight, and we wondered how it would end. The policy in Gorongosa was not to interfere with the course of nature, and any suffering injured animal was simply left to manage as best it could. A doubtful policy from the humane point of view, but possibly a sound one in the light of the theory that only the fittest survive, the rest becoming prey to natural predators, thus fulfilling the laws of Nature which were in operation many hundreds of millions of years before man was thought of.

CHAPTER 5

The Reluctant Bull

On returning from a holiday there should be ample time allowed to recover from it; it is uncivilized in the extreme to begin work the moment one returns. One's performance cannot be good if one is plunged too rapidly from one world to another.

These thoughts were uppermost in my mind while we drove the last lap home after our idyllic two weeks in Gorongosa. The nearer to White River we came, the louder became my inward protestations; until my mind, somewhat clouded by that morning's breakfast celebrations (for it was Howard's birthday), became a drumming, pounding, throbbing headache with only one aim in mind: "Never to work again, and to cease at once to be a public servant."

Such trends of thought are always quickly dispelled as soon as I walk into my house. It matters not whether I have been absent for one week or two months: the telephone rings and rings with the same insistent, maddening, impatient sound. This afternoon of my return was no exception. As so often happens, the first call I took after any holiday brought me down to earth with a bump; and in a way this is almost therapeutic – it gives me no time to cherish further thoughts about giving up my career.

"Is that you, Doctor?"

"Yes, it is," I answered regretfully, very tempted to say that the doctor was still away on holiday. "Can I help you?"

"This is Petronella Mix speaking. Doctor, I have a sex problem."

"I am afraid you have the wrong number," I said with some relief. "Please hang on whilst I get you the number of the human doctor. I only attend to animal problems."

"But Doctor," said the pleading voice in alarm, "this *is* an animal problem. My sex is perfectly all right, but my tom cat seems all mixed up. He had kittens a few days ago, seven of them, but I can assure you that until then he was definitely male. Do you think he might have undergone a sex-change?"

At this point my sense of humour reasserted itself and I began to enjoy this quite ridiculous conversation. "I doubt that there has been a sex-change, though of course, it is not impossible. I am afraid nothing can be done now, and you have abundant proof that your tom cat is a female. I don't think there is anything I can do for you."

"Oh, Doctor, but there is, there is!" The dear lady was getting desperate. "I want you to come out to the farm at once and sex the kittens so that this sort of thing can never happen again. You see, I have become the laughing-stock of the family, for everyone says that it must be the first time that Caesar had kittens."

"Why don't you re-christen her Cleopatra?" I suggested weakly, for my children, picking up scraps of the conversation, were in hysterics.

"I'll do as you suggest," said the lady cheerfully, "and I would be so grateful if you would come out and sex my other cats too. I have twenty-seven altogether and if I know when you are coming, I'll see that they are all at home."

So I made a date and replaced the receiver and thanked my lucky stars that this sort of problem was a rarity. My children, however, were determined to make the most of this fascinating conversation, and settled down to quiz me. "What is a sex-change, Mummy?" asked my little son; "and why was the lady so upset about having kittens?" My daughter, aged eight, replied with great authority. "Ladies do not have kittens, Guy, it was the tom cat that had them. Mummy told her to change his name so that the kittens would have a mother; that's what is called a sex-change." I left them to go and unpack, too exhausted to go into further explanations; time later to sort out the intricacies of this side of life!

That afternoon as I was re-gathering the reins of my household and practice, musing upon the events of the past weeks, another incident floated into my consciousness. This had occurred the year before, and had been equally puzzling and nonsensical.

It had been Christmas time, and life had taken on a holiday atmosphere, even though work continued as before. In the midst of a Christmas dinner-party the phone had rung, and I answered, hoping against hope that this was not a far-away calving case, or an overdue Caesarian section. In actual fact it was a very distressed old lady who had an enormous grievance which she wanted me to sort out at once, at that very moment. "I am reporting a case of cruelty to you"; she spoke with a voice of one used to command. "I want you to come out at once and see to it. I will meet you at the bottom of the drive." Not a word as to who she was, where she lived, or what the cause of her energetic complaint. After much questioning I finally discovered that a cow, grazing on the slopes above her farmstead, wore a bell about her neck which the complainant insisted was a dreadful torture. It had all come to a head when the police and the local S.P.C.A. had refused to take action. I was, in fact, her last hope, and she was absolutely certain that I would help her. I made it clear that I did not consider cowbells cruel, that they had been worn by European bovines for hundreds of years. She at once became offensive and belligerent, and accused me of being an accessory to cruelty. My reply however, silenced her. "Unless you are a cow yourself," I said as mildly as I could, "you cannot judge whether the wearing of a bell is disturbing or not. I cannot help you any further, so a merry Christmas to you, and a peaceful New Year." "Merry Christmas to you too, Doctor." The old lady sounded almost subdued and finally abandoned me as a hopeless case. For some time afterwards I heard murmurings and rumours in the district about an imminent court case, in which the plaintiff was to be the lady of the cowbell; and if this case actually reached the courts it would surprise me hardly at all: the tireless energy of our above-fifty female population is both amazing and endless. A very few of these pillars of society are still endowed with husbands, having usually outlived them by twenty or thirty years. Has this occurred because, being more active, and having the energy derived from spirit, these ladies have never really aged except in physical appearance? Or is it because their men, worn out with trying to keep up with their wives, have just laid down their heads in despair? Whatever the truth of it, we have much to learn from this generation of stayers, born in the last half of the nineteenth century.

The Lowveld Show was about to begin. As an annual event it drew together the inhabitants of the central and outlying districts, even attracting entries from the Highveld cities. During its three-day period, which gave scope to everything from sugar-candy stalls to first-class equestrian events, the entire population met and mingled on the dry and dusty showground, usually at the windiest part of the year, in the winter months.

You could take your pick. There was everything to be seen: the needlework your child did at school, chickens, prize citrus and sub-tropical fruit displays laid in spectacular and expert manner, fortune tellers, police dogs, merry-go-rounds, ribald paintings. The stock section was usually well filled, the horse events the main attraction. From the big city came the show-followers with their groomed hunters and their suave, over-groomed riders who took prize after prize from the locals. From territory to the east came smooth, electric, hot-blooded steeds mastered by cavalry officers of the same temperament. It was all very well organised; one event followed another with smooth rhythm, and there were very few mishaps. Some of the Lowveld bachelors – stalwart helpers from the beginning of time – controlled the jumps, kept law and order, and added colour to life in general by their curious and endearing appearance, more or less eccentric. Over the loud-speakers incessant calls could be heard, and a whirr of mechanical devices filled the background, coming from the agricultural section. This drew a great number of farmers; even if too poor to purchase these fantastic vehicles and motorised devices for speedy and economical farming, they loved to spend hours having them explained and demonstrated, thus satisfying that curiosity, that basic boyish love for such toys that no man ever loses.

Together with two other veterinarians, I took turn to do duty in case of trouble. It meant staying at the Show for two half days whiling away the time with old friends whom I saw only once a year, drinking pints of ghastly coffee, inspecting the stalls in minute detail until I knew them by heart, and attending to the odd case which might occur and need immediate attention. On this particular opening day of the umpteenth Lowveld Show, I was idly watching the colourful noisy crowd over a cup of that un-drinkable coffee, when I heard my name called over the loud-speaker. "Please come to the stock-judging section at once. Please come at once, you are badly needed."

I leapt to my feet, took leave of my friends, and moved as fast as

I could without losing my dignity. On the way I had to brush off the over-eager How-to-Cook-American-Rice-Best lady demonstrator, who wanted me to know that I would feel much better if I ate my rice cooked the proper way. I also had a near collision with the Singer sewing-machine stall, which looked as if it would collapse at any moment – in fact, I did not dare look back in case the stall had collapsed after my impact with it. At last I reached the ring in a breathless state, and was met by an equally breathless farmer who had been trying to bring to life his champion Jersey bull without success. A cluster of sympathetic farmers at first blocked my view, and I wondered what was going on. One had his teeth buried in the unfortunate's tail, the next was pouring water in the ears, while the rest cursed and encouraged in turn. The spectators and judges stood back and watched the scene with obvious relish. "Make way for the doc." The crowd parted and let me through. "I think he must be ill, doc. He was all right, and I was sure he was going to win his class, when suddenly he just lay down, and we can't get him up."

In spite of constant man-handling, the bull, twitching his moist nose in contempt, refused to move or even to react to the treatment in the slightest. I carefully examined him, took his temperature and checked his heart; but all the time, from his very attitude, I could see that there was nothing medically wrong with him. He had been led round and round the ring for over an hour and being an intelligent sort of bull, he had just gone on strike. "Your bull is all right. Tell everyone to clear the ring, and fetch some lucerne and a bowl of dairy cubes." When the ring was clear of humanity, and the bull saw the food being brought, he at once arose and moved to the fodder and contentedly munched, quite unaware of the commotion he had caused. After that there was no more trouble, and I was delighted that the farmers – often very sceptical of new ideas and even more so when these are presented to them by a female – admitted gratefully that I had put my finger on the trouble at once. "Never thought that cattle were clever or felt a thing. Trust a woman to work that one out. No man could ever have that much reason. Must be instinct, a woman's instinct."

Yes, indeed, a woman's instinct is a blessing to us and amazingly useful in veterinary work. So very often our cases are enigmatic and cannot be solved by ordinary means of diagnosis. In such a case what does a man do? Guess a little, blunder a little, hope for the best. A woman vet, of course, does the same, but the mystery of some cases resolves itself if she will allow her intuition to come into play. Perhaps it is an uncertain, uncanny, and even dangerous way of practising; yet the proof of the pudding lies in the eating, and there have been many cases in my professional career when I would have done well to stand by my first strong impression, rather than allow my reason to take over and lead me astray.

As I was leaving the stock-section to seek out my friends, avoiding at all cost the Cook-Rice-the-American-Way lady, I again heard my name called, but this time by an African. I immediately recognized him as the driver of one of my Jersey-herd clients, who in this case was also the owner of a fabulous estate, the most magnificent gardens for hundreds of miles, a swarm of poodles (only the collective noun 'swarm' can satisfy as description of this nest of curly-haired horrors), and a grand home with priceless *objets d'art* with an eastern flavour. She was also the employer of many farm managers and farm hands, among them a fierce ex-land-girl who nursed and loved and cared for the cattle.

It was the latter who was now in need of help; and although her problem was indeed a human one, I was still called upon to help, being the only person – or so the employer thought – who was not only familiar with the antics of animals but also with those of the animals' keeper. My friend was beside herself with worry, for her cow-girl appeared to be suffering from a bad attack of nerves, and threatened at any moment to sink out of circulation rather like the Jersey bull. But while the latter went calmly on strike in the full possession of his mental processes, the former could not control herself either physically or mentally, and was in imminent danger of collapse.

As I approached the ring, which was crowded with spectators, I could see Enid swaying at the side of a really beautiful, silky-coated Jersey heifer, which gave the impression that she was leading the lady rather than the other way about. As Enid spotted me, she let go the halter and stumbled to the side, a piteous sight, with tears streaming down her face. She was perilously close to a complete nervous breakdown, and I felt it was of vital importance that she should leave the ring and rest, so as to avert a catastrophe. A substitute was quickly found for her, and while she was being comforted by her boss in the back of a hay-scented cow-stall, I rushed to the village to obtain some tranquillising drug as quickly as possible. There was no time to consult a doctor or worry about etiquette; something had to be done, and clearly I was the one who had to do it. Praying that I would not be needed in the next half-hour, I drove full-speed and managed to return without incident, being admitted by the entrance keeper, who was shaking his head and muttering about mad woman drivers as I passed. Within an hour our cow-girl was as good as new; in an artificial state, certainly, but nevertheless, this was an effective remedy for her attack of the jitters, and she managed to hold her own very well for the next three days, without anyone being any the wiser.

It was interesting that a very wild and intractable bull, aptly named Rocket, who was under her care, had to be tranquillised by injection with the same substance for two days before and until three days after the end of the Show. Without the aid of this sedation, it would have been impossible to control him.

I think very few doctors realise how similar are the conditions which we have to contend with in veterinary medicine, and how parallel are the treatments which are applied. It is often just a matter of different dosage and of different resistance to certain drugs; on the whole the animal kingdom has more resilience, and the reactions and allergies which human patients suffer from are very rare indeed.

I had been attending the poodle tribe for years. Mrs. Somer was a delightful person who surrounded herself with only the best, and who did not stint her animals anything. She could not, however, prevent herself from becoming a typical poodle-mistress, marked as such by her subservience to her pets. In such a household the days are planned around the dogs; and when these become sick, which frequently happens, the day's routine is woven around their needs. Unlike others who can well afford expensive antibiotics when these become necessary but refuse to spend their wealth on a mere dog, this lady could not do enough for her canines, and it was a pleasure to attend to them. Poodles are always difficult patients, and so the pleasure is not without its drawbacks. These drawbacks are, in a way, connected with their great intelligence; for once they have tasted medicine they will disappear not merely when they see the bottle and spoon appear,

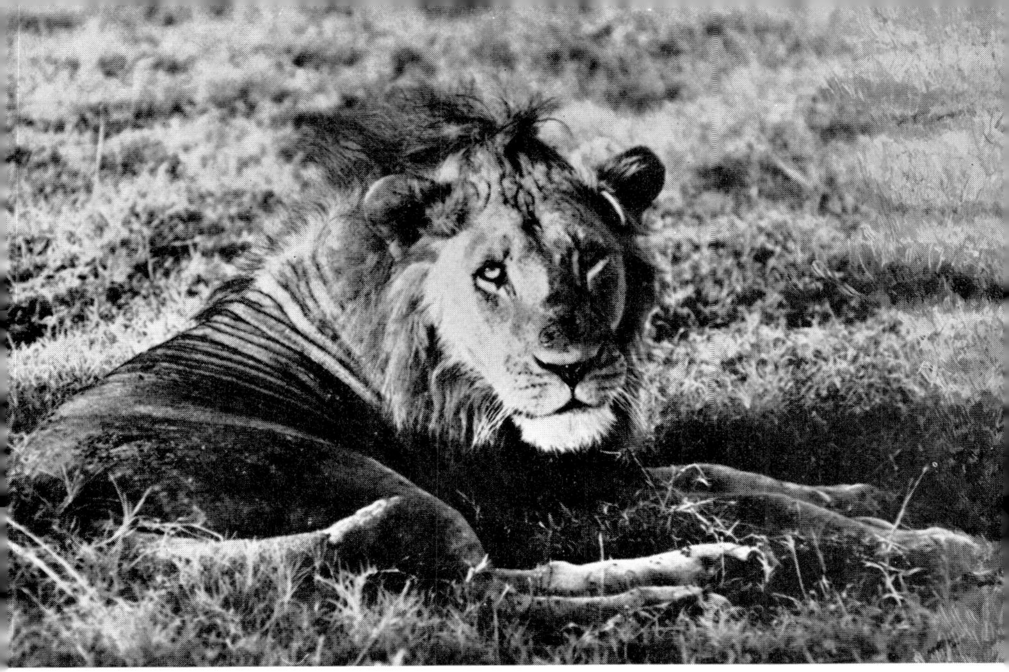

4. Chico, the tailless lion.

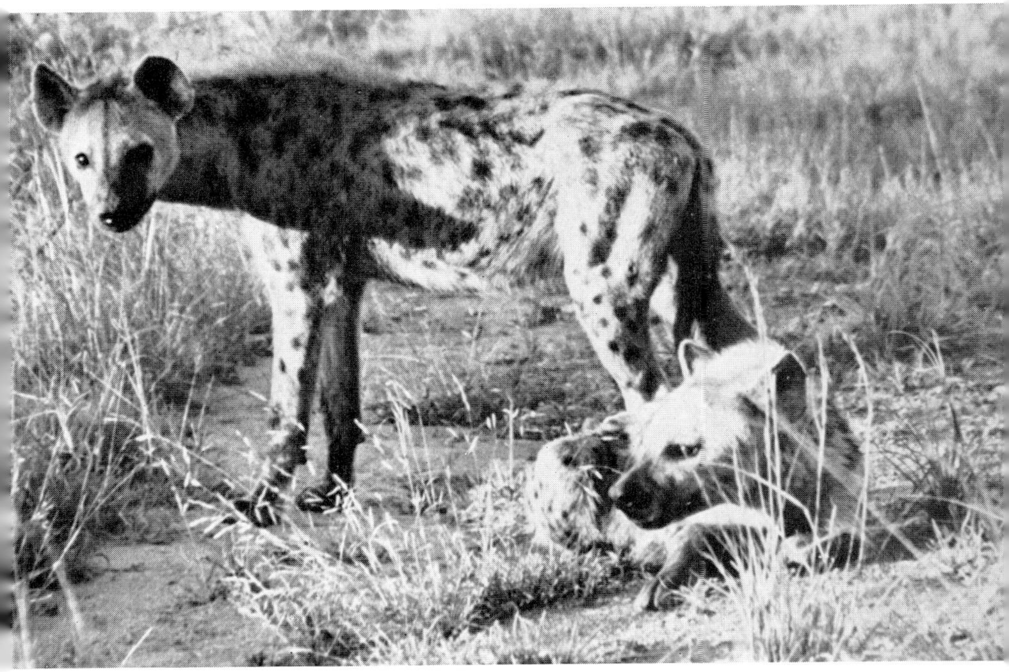

5. Hyenas waiting their turn.

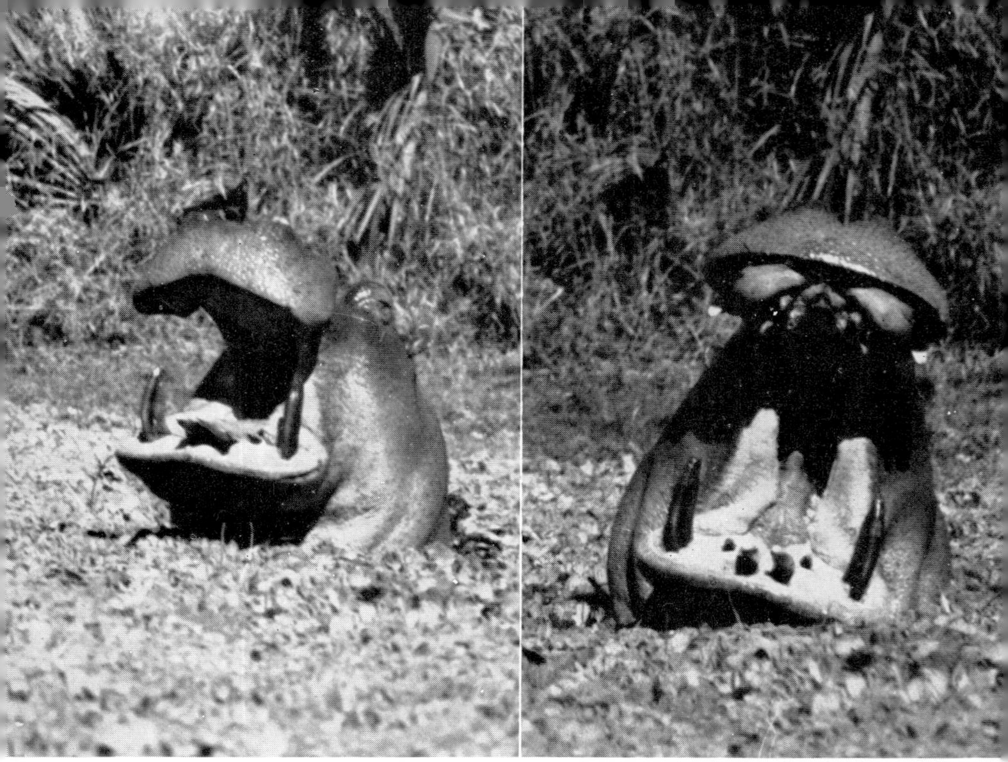

6. Ioâo, the hermit hippo, giving an unforgettable view of his tonsils.

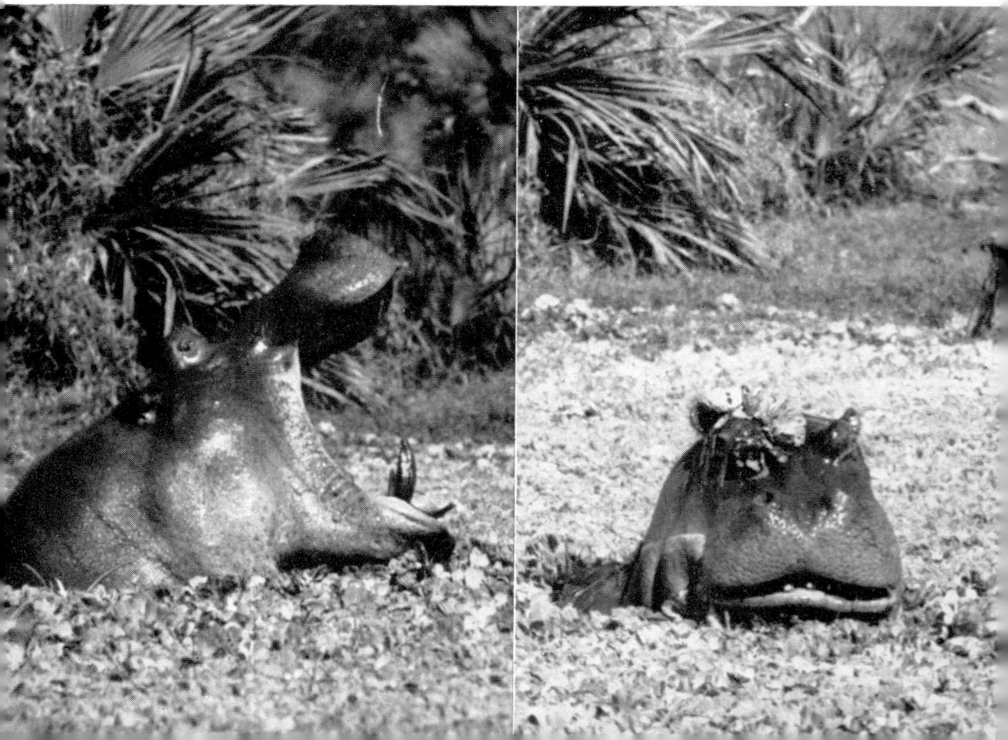

but before that; they will quietly retire to some inaccessible spot every four or six hours, whenever they know they are about to be dosed. The process of giving them their medicine is in no way an easy one, for they clench their little jaws as firmly as any bull-terrier, and some acquire the art of holding the liquid in their cheeks until it is safe to spit it out.

Quite apart from all these joys, they react violently to certain drugs and procedures, this being partly due to their inbred and often neurotic natures, and partly to the fact that they work themselves into a state of apprehensive frenzy whenever they approach a veterinarian's consulting-rooms.

These poodles, led by the inimitable patriarch Grock, who seemed to have sired practically every poodle in the district over the past ten years, were continuously plagued by attacks of tonsillitis, of which there seemed to be no end. Finally, in despair, I decided to operate and remove countless poodle-tonsils which seemed to have become infected beyond repair. After this, there was a time during which there was no sickness or feeding trouble, and my visits to the farm were confined to cattle-attendance – always followed by a delicious breakfast when the work was done. This state of affairs did not last, however. Within a few months the black, grey and white aristocrats developed a new disease, which proved to be lifelong and only curable for periods at a time: they all developed an itch. But this was no ordinary itch, for it seemed to have no cause whatsoever. The usual skin infections, external and internal parasites, and dietary deficiences were all absent here; I came to the unwilling conclusion that these were cases of self-inflicted neurosis, replacing the previous tonsil episode in a collective effort to continue to draw attention to themselves. I may be harsh in this judgement, but it is not impossible; in highly intelligent animals even a subconscious reaction such as this is not unusual.

Now the same agonies began all over again; but this time the dogs, which slept on their mistress's bed, caused her endless sleepless nights, for they never ceased their scratching and grunting. The treatments helped only within limits and for a time. I was full of admiration for Mrs. Somer; she continued to dose her beloved canines when most people would have had them destroyed. She spared neither energy nor money, and did not stint them in any way. Nor did she blame me when the treatment brought little relief, except for brief periods; she simply accepted the inevitable with her usual patient smile, in spite of the fact that at this time she was a very ill woman herself.

When she died, her poodle tribe was dispersed all over the Lowveld; and perhaps the consequent mingling with new blood and type will help to eliminate the inherent weaknesses which seemed to worsen with each new litter born. I had to destroy old Grock myself in the end; my thought, as his tough little body went limp, was for Mrs. Somer; I hoped that if her dog joined her in heaven he would treat her with more consideration.

CHAPTER 6

Even a Mouse . . .

One of the great joys of country practice is the immense and never-ending variety of one's clientele; yesterday the sufferings of an inbred poodle, today the robust earthiness of farm animals, and tomorrow, perhaps, the human animal. One moment I was lost in the Sabie mountains, searching for a forestry logging mule which had injured its foot, seemingly a moment later I found myself grappling with a problem that was, strictly speaking, outside the veterinary curriculum – though I have often felt that this side of our teaching was much neglected.

Choosing the soundest specimen for reproduction purposes is quite an everyday business, but the problem of helping a human female in the choice of her next husband posed rather an unveterinary problem, though the basic principles seem to be closely related. I had just descended from an early morning visit to a high pine plantation, and had watched the early morning mists, which lay draped over the valley like a bridal veil, disperse and drift and disappear into threads of nothingness as the rising sun pierced the chill air. From the vantage point of a rust-lichen covered rock I had witnessed yet another dawn unfold, enjoying my thermos of coffee for as long as I dared stay out of contact between calls. During those moments I felt myself merged into the world of silence, almost resenting the work which drew me down again, away from the dreamland of endless pine-forests and the scent of wild mushrooms.

It was easy to recognise Mrs. van Wert, for she stood among a flurry of dogs of divers shapes and sizes, leaning upon her bicycle, her knitting trailing beside her, busy even at this early hour. There was no doubt of her identity: already at the corner of my street I could see the lady, dumpy shaped frizzy hair, her dogs about her as though protecting their mistress from the chill morning breeze. I unlocked the door and invited her in, relieved that she had come so early; her visits usually created mild havoc in the waiting-room, since she insisted on bringing her means of transport inside, worried that some passing *piccanin* (African young boy) might make off with it. Apart from this, her dogs had a most belligerent nature, and when in company created a common front, forgetting their own differences and attacking any other animal in sight with gusto. Her visits always occurred twice weekly, for she believed in taking great care of her canines – far greater care, in fact, than she took of herself. The chow-cross bitch was running to fat, and began to scratch herself unceasingly whenever the temperature rose above 70 degrees Fahrenheit. For some reason her owner called her Dreamgirl, a strange name considering that she must have been a nightmare to sleep with. The two black dogs, Darling and Thunder, vied for her affections; with the result that both were constantly thin and out of breath. These explanations did not satisfy their doting mistress and I was forced to make regular examinations for internal parasites, to make sure that neither of them had worms. All this took a great deal of time, but I could not refuse to see this foursome: if I asked her to come back another time, it would certainly be on an even busier day.

"You are very early, Mrs. van Wert; having more trouble?" While I braced myself to listen to the usual history, which normally lasted about ten minutes, my mind was turning over the previous case; and I found myself wondering why the forestry manager I had just visited had waited so long before calling me in. The mule's foot I had examined had already turned very septic. Lost in this reverie, I was still able to take in the gist of the conversation, and so I suddenly brought my mind into sharp focus. It seemed that her pets had come along just for the run, and that the object of her visit was primarily to seek my help in a matrimonial matter. It appeared that this amazing woman, who had been married twice before and divorced twice, had acquired both her previous husbands by advertisements in the matrimonial columns; now, once again, she was busily engaged in dealing with the replies to a third such advertisement. There were no less than twenty-five applications, most of whom had supplied photographs; these, I thought, might be very misleading, as some had obviously been taken thirty years or so previously. "Oh, Doctor

Sue," she pleaded, "you know so much about breeding and good stock. I do so want to marry a really good and handsome and rich and kind man this time, one who is sure to let *all* the dogs sleep in bed with us. My last husband – can you believe it? – divorced me on the grounds that our bed was always flea-ridden! What a lot of nonsense, you can see for yourself how clean the little darlings are!"

Wonder upon wonders: if only my old Professor of Medicine could have seen me at that moment. He had always said that women have the most colourful practices, since they attract such a variety of problems.

By this time my secretary had arrived and was trying very hard to keep a straight face. She did not have to try very long, for Mrs. van Wert preferred to keep this conversation tête à tête, and the door was discreetly closed. While tea was being brewed, I studied those fascinating photographs. "You can have the one you like *second* best." I was somewhat startled by this remark; it had not occurred to me that I also figured in this scheme. "You should not stay alone, you know, Doctor Sue"; Mrs. van Wert was the kindest person imaginable, and she was determined to find a man for me too, though she reminded me gently that the first choice would always be hers.

I managed to distract her from this line of thought, and after about half an hour – by which time I knew most intimately the deepest thoughts of her would-be husbands – I chose for her a very handsome young-looking man, a Canadian pilot, whose letters seemed a little more realistic, but yet contained the essence of romance which is proper on such an occasion. By the time the husband-huntress had left my rooms, we had made a choice mutually pleasing, and I had also helped her to reply to some of the unsuccessful applications. I was now quite excited about this venture, waiting for the day when the husband-to-be would be brought to me for inspection, as she had threatened. Unfortunately all these attempts to settle into blissful domesticity failed her for the time being; she had, after all, not listened to my advice to be diplomatic and somewhat reserved, and had unwisely sent a telegram to the young airman which had read like this: "Please come quickly to see me, there are others waiting to be looked at." Two weeks after sending this disastrous message, she received a reply:

"Sorry, cannot bear to stand in queues." So it all started again – the letters to the papers, the ardent hopeful replies, the photograph selection, the breathless waiting. Finally Mrs. van Wert left the district to go and 'look some over' and was never heard of there again; we missed her and feared for her, hoping that the sweetness of her nature and her absolute trust and childishness would not get her into irreparable trouble.

Although I enjoyed my small-animal work immensely, at certain times of the year, particularly in winter, my practice became a sort of dog-and-cat circus. The rains and the heat produced an environment which was an ideal breeding-ground for ticks and other external and internal parasites, and these thrived and battened unmercifully upon the ovine, equine and bovine stock. In the Lowveld there is a saying which is most appropriate: "In summer the ticks and mosquitoes eat us, but in winter our visitors consume us." Small wonder that our friends flocked down to us in the cooler season, for our climate from April to August was a succession of glorious warm days and crisp clear nights. The monotony of the small-animal work was broken by the advent of city dwellers – some friends, some acquaintances, often family. I left them very much to their own devices, as I was usually busy with the practice: alternatively, I roped them into helping me, which they usually enjoyed immensely – particularly their children, who almost always developed a longing to become veterinarians (to their parents' horror) during this holiday period.

Autumn (April in Southern Africa) marked the beginning of the spaying season: suddenly the whole district, which stretched one hundred miles in each direction, became aware of the fact that its pets were possessed of sexual characteristics and prowess, and their owners rushed to the surgery to put this right at once. At the end of such a season, I always felt that every single small animal in the area was now devoid of sex, and yet each year the new generation presented itself at my door with never-failing regularity. It would be an understatement to say that this type of work is soulless. It is truer to call it soul-destroying, especially as the principle involved is very questionable. Animals that are desexed in maturity sometimes lose much of their zest in life, especially male felines, who end up as miserable bundles of fur, living a semi-frustrated life without knowing what it is they are missing.

It was during one of these winter periods, about the time when Mrs. van Wert had relieved my boredom with her unusual request, that a certain young man came to me, blushing and hesitant, quite unable to bring to the surface what he had come to say until he had been strengthened with three strong cups of coffee. "Doctor," he stammered, "I want you to spay Jenny for me, but I want you to do it in a special way so that she can go on having fun." A bespectacled maiden lady, waiting for her pet to recover a little from the anaesthetic, looked up, shocked out of her reverie. "I am afraid that the operation we usually perform is somewhat different from the human one." The young farmer was biting his nails in distress by this time, and the waiting lady had shrunk back into her seat, as though trying to disappear altogether. "You must know exactly what it is you are asking," I continued, "for though women do not lose their sex-appeal when ovaro-hysterectomised, this is exactly the opposite of what we hope will happen to the canine. It is that very sex-appeal which, if retained, is the sure cause of sleepless nights and court cases between neighbours." "I see." Ted Bachelor seemed to be thinking this over very carefully, and then summed up superhuman courage before he spoke again. "I want Jenny to have fun, like people do. Please don't worry about our neighbours: the nearest one is twenty miles away, anyway. Just as long as she doesn't have puppies."

And so it was settled for the following week; I felt much better about mankind after that, for although there are only a very few who really care for their animals, one instance like this seemed to offset the thoughtlessness of the many. This was to be a month of sex problems; in my practice, cases of similar type tended to follow one upon another, and at the end of this period I felt almost ready to set up as a sex-expert. Almost: I still had vivid memories of being unmercifully ragged by fellow students when I was apparently the most naïve and unknowledgeable student in our whole year, which numbered a hundred and ten. Even at the outset of my veterinary career in the African Lowveld, I seemed to be devoid of some of the experience that a vet is expected to possess, and for many years I could not live down an incident which occurred on my first visit to the Kruger National Park. My friend, Howard Kirk, a great authority on wild life and a wonderful guide, showed me my first giraffe, an enormous dark-patterned animal which towered over us from the side of the road. "He has a hernia, poor old chap," I commented, and was rather surprised that Howard did not even utter a word of sympathy at the giraffe's terrible plight but drove on for some time in complete silence. Very soon we came across more giraffe, this time in a group of six, browsing among the acacia trees; they were so near that we could see them curl their tongues for food, draw it back into their mouth, chew from side to side in what appeared to be a rotary motion, and swallow the resultant bolus while already looking for the next tit-bit. "Look Sue, they all have hernias!" I was startled to see that each of the six giants had indeed the appearance of the first, and for a moment I was completely nonplussed. As the truth dawned on me I heard the soft laughter of my companion and realised that, once more, I had laid myself wide open. "I don't think I'll ever bring my animals to you for de-sexing; you might try to spay my male ridgeback!"

After eight years I was still reminded of this each time we visited the park, for the very idea that a vet did not know the external sexual characteristics of any animal amused everyone intensely. The only excuse I had, though it did not carry much weight, was that we had never been instructed in the anatomy of wild animals. The male giraffe is certainly oddly arranged. It was fortunate that no hyena required to be sexed at that time, for I was not even aware of the fact that this animal is the most difficult of all to sex, and that the young hyena has in fact no external sexual dimorphism at all. I had heard it said that hyenas are bisexual, but I had passed this by as an old wives' tale: it was too difficult to believe. On a later occasion, visiting a Zululand sanctuary, I met a tame hyena, only a few months old, at the home of one of the rangers; he himself did not know what sex his sharp-jawed, incredibly strong-muscled pet was. Fortunately, a veterinarian from East Africa was present, an expert on these matters; he explained to us the strange and most unusual formation of sexual organs in these animals, as far as it is known. The normally accepted pattern of development has certainly by-passed these carnivorous scavengers, and there is much research yet to be done on this species.

It was a morning of surprises. An African youth, who had been hovering near the door for some time, was asked by my secretary to bring in his "animal sick in the tail". He promptly did so, presenting a fully grown Jerusalem ass, which took an intense dislike to my instrument cabinet, and demonstrated this by endeavouring to kick its glass front to pieces. The youth, smiling apologetically, remarked ingratiatingly that perhaps *Inbongolo* (Zulu for Donkey) did not feel quite at home, and perhaps I would be kind enough to give a *jova* (injection) to make him feel calmer. As I was determined to effect the ass's departure as soon as possible, I could not agree with this suggestion, since the patient might have bedded down in my operating-examination room for several hours. We therefore blindfolded him and led him back outside where, to the delight of numerous and mostly related Bantu who had come to see the fun, I lanced an abscess at the base of the tail, trying to keep my dignity and professional demeanour while working on the sidewalk with the crowd cheering my every move. "I prefer to make payment now, Doctor, how much *mali* (money) is it?" "Five shillings." "Ow, so little," whistled one of the bystanders. "We will bring you all our oxen and mules too." Which they often did, sometimes to my town surgery, or else I would find some enormous, truculent black ox tied to my tree early in the morning, or a skeleton-thin, mange-ridden dog left tied to the door, with a note: "Will return soon, please make better." The owner always did return, but as time means nothing to the Bantu, the dog would usually remain in my kennels (if it survived) for a month or two at least. The native then might return one fine day out of nowhere, having probably walked for fifty miles to reach me; and after making polite inquiries about my health, and after being strengthened by some bread and coffee, he would then tentatively ask after his dog. If the dog had improved there would be great joy and the demonstration of affection was by no means one-sided; these dogs adored their masters and often showed animosity towards a white skin, as also happened in reverse.

Breathing a sigh of relief as the ass disappeared down the street, I returned to my rooms to find an Afrikaans farmer (Afrikaaners are of Dutch descent, early settlers in South Africa) who had been patiently waiting for some time, smoking his pipe, seemingly occupied with his own thoughts, unaware of the turmoil around him. I recognised him as a typical Lowvelder, a hard-working and kindly, philosophical, weatherbeaten, speaking only broken English without holding any resentment for someone like myself who spoke only broken Afrikaans. Dressed in khaki trousers, khaki shirt and *veldskoene* (rough ankle-high working boots), his bush hat on his knees, he remained almost immobile while I dashed in and out. My African orderly was, with his usual quiet efficiency, boiling up instruments for the next operation: this was to be an amputation of the hind leg of a Great Dane dog, who had been caught in a vicious gin-trap, no doubt set for a buck. Used instruments were being washed, the tea kettle was on the boil, and then into the midst of this burst a mob of children, including my own, who had managed to get passes for break-time and had come to see if anything of interest was going on. My daughter gave them a conducted tour of the premises with pride, explaining everything in great detail, while Sam (the orderly) looked on benevolently, seeing that no harm would come either to them or to his patient. When the distant school bell was heard, the accompanying exodus was no small relief, for I was already two hours behind my schedule.

Tea had been poured for everyone present, and Sam came to fill his cup. I used the time for writing up the case cards while the details were still fresh in my memory. The farmer continued to sit introspectively, enjoying his tea; after some moments I joined him, inquiring what I could do for him. "You lady, nothing at all", he replied pleasantly, "it's the *veearts* (vet) I have come to see. When will he be back?" I was completely taken aback: I thought the district would be aware of my sex by this time. I should have realised that some of the outlying farmers, who rarely come into the village, had little contact with new developments; often, as I learnt later, they sought the advice of one of the chemists, who would usually refer them to me if the case was beyond their tackling. "There's a new vet in the district." And that was all, though I suspect that they withheld further particulars just for the fun of it, knowing full well how old-fashioned some of the backveld farmers were.

"*Dit is ek, ek is regtig die veearts* (It is I, I am really the vet)." "Oo." The farmer rose in his chair, grabbed his hat, and began to back away, blushing even through his tanned face to the base of his open collar. In a flash it dawned upon me that this poor man had no ordinary problem and that the advice he sought must have concerned some aspect of reproduction, the last thing he would have discussed with a woman. "Please sit down and have some more tea. I am sure I can help you." And so, slowly and surely he warmed to the subject, between answering my questions concerning his crops, his children, his neighbourhood, hardly aware that his horror at the thought of divulging a sex problem was melting away. This all took precious time, yet the winning over of this section of the community was a challenge to me. Being a woman, I was driven with feminine obstinacy to prove that I could, indeed, practise among all kinds of people, and so defeat the pessimism of my former colleagues, who had held no hope for my survival, either professionally or physically, in country practice.

"It's my bull, he can't do it." I had guessed this was the problem, but had known better than to forestall his statement. "Lady, maybe you can't understand me, you see, he's been all right for years and had good calves, and now, suddenly, he just, well, he just cannot *do* it. There seems to be something wrong with his, his . . . well, lady, his navel. Could you come out and have a look at it?" Poor man, I suffered with him, for this interview was obviously something of an ordeal. "Please don't worry, Meneer," I soothed, "many bulls have this sort of trouble. We will have to throw the bull to have a good look at his navel, so please see there is plenty of help when I come out."

And indeed, there was a tremendous turn out when I did arrive a few afternoons later with my small daughter, who had been visiting a neighbouring farm. The whole family was there, from the great-grandfather down to the latest arrivals. As happened often, they had all come to witness the fiesta, and to see a woman perform on a bull was as good as a circus. They had collected all their cow-hide *rims* (ropes) and were ready to throw the poor beast by tripping his legs, as is usually done. I waved them firmly away, placed my own rope upon the bull while he was being held by the nose, and directed three of the men to pull the free end backwards in a straight line (Reuff's method) while one held the head. This simple procedure resulted in the immediate and total collapse of the animal, without snort or kick, within a matter of half a minute; there was a reaction from the bystanders which indicated that had all this taken place a hundred years ago, I would have surely been burnt at the stake as a witch.

The rest of the case was simple; an infection of the "waterworks", as my daughter loudly called it to the embarrassment of the inhibited onlookers, had clearly been the cause of impotence, and this would respond to a wide-spectrum antibiotic. I was fortunate to be successful in this case, for once these good people were convinced that I could cure their animals' ills, they called me in regularly and became excellent clients, showing their appreciation in many touching ways, such as paying their accounts regularly (very rare indeed among the English Lowveld population) and keeping me constantly supplied with fresh fruit and vegetables. I had been warned that as I was an Englishwoman this section of the farming community would never accept me, however good I might be. This warning, fortunately proved to be groundless, and in the end my practice had a large Afrikaans following, and some became my good friends in the course of time.

This month of strange case-records with an accent on sex includes one which was so ludicrous that I lost my composure completely and frightened away a client, a sin beyond sin among vets! He was a small bewhiskered man, paunchy, aggressive and beady-eyed; the air around him was so tinged with the aroma of brandy that at first I mistook his question for an alcoholic joke. "Doc, will you castrate my mouse?" I laughed out loud, told him that he needed a circus vet, and asked him what he had really come for. "It's true. This mouse is causing me a lot of trouble and soon the whole house will be overrun. I'll pay anything for the operation, but if you cannot do it, I'll go somewhere else." "I'll have to use a lens or a microscope," I said, "and then there is the difficulty about the anaesthetic. I will have to consult my books." I am afraid I could not take this case too seriously and the little man sensed, perhaps, that he was being made a fool of. He suddenly leapt up, stared at me defiantly, and blurted out: "I wouldn't let you castrate my mouse if you begged me. I'll go where there is a man for the job. Women shouldn't meddle with sex anyway."

EVEN A MOUSE . ..

The cave-man outlook over again, and this time perhaps not a bad thing, for no good can ever come of meddling with the sex-life of a mouse.

While I was recovering from the surprise of the mouse-man, feeling that perhaps I had let my profession down a little with my unladylike behaviour, the telephone rang and I decided to take this call which was paged as urgent, and wait until the afternoon to perform a planned amputation. "My name is Reilly, I am warden of the Sabie Sand Game Sanctuary. I have a leopard who is getting to *like* children too much, so would you spay her please? As soon as possible?" "Lady," interrupted the White River exchange, "are you finished?" "I haven't even started, please don't cut us off." "All right, lady," the exchange concurred, sourly, "hurry up". "Hello, hello, is that you, Doctor, did you hear what I said? I want you to spay my leopard, Lulu, she is only eight months old." "Please give me your number so I can call you back. I will have to consult my engagement book." This wasn't entirely true, since in actual fact I wanted some breathing space and some time to consider the enormity of this request. It is one thing to spay a domestic cat, but to tackle a wild leopard who might not appreciate such interference was quite another thing. I therefore telephoned the Professor of Surgery at the Veterinary Institution at Onderstepoort, two hundred and fifty miles away, to seek advice. This surgeon was a good friend and had always given me much help in the past years, even taking on cases which I felt I should not, or could not attempt myself. He offered to perform the operation with me in his own department, saying that he would keep the leopard for the vital recuperative period afterwards. Having made this arrangement, I could now look forward to this unusual case with pleasurable anticipation.

Perhaps the sequel to this, sad though it was, turned out for the best. Terry Reilly did not want to give Lulu to a zoo, and he knew that release would not ensure her survival; but she was becoming very dangerous to everyone except her owner. It is doubtful whether spaying would have subdued her temperament. I learnt later that she had died one week after that long-distance conversation while on active service with her beloved boss, who was doing the rounds of his extensive domain. A wildebeest had suddenly charged across the track and Terry, in trying to avoid it, had managed only to manoeuvre the Land-Rover into a tree; he saved the life of the gnu but was unable to prevent damage to himself, Lulu and the vehicle. His dog, the venerable Simba, escaped unhurt, but Terry remained unconscious for some hours and Lulu, also concussed, did not ever regain consciousness again. It was not for several months that I met Terry Reilly in the flesh; from that time on we became closely associated, since our paths often crossed in our different spheres of similar work – conservation and care of animal life.

CHAPTER 7

Zebra in the Mist

About one year later I discovered more about Lulu. I had not guessed that she had been adopted at such an early age; one could have expected her to be more amenable to strangers since she had known the human touch for so long. But it is well-known that leopards are difficult to tame; few people – notably Ralph Helfer of 'Africa U.S.A.' near Los Angeles – have ever managed to make the handling of these big cats possible and safe. A leopard-farmer in Southern Africa had the terrible experience of seeing his daughter mauled by a familiar and hitherto friendly leopard, while the scene was being filmed. I had heard of several similar cases; and although I had always wanted to possess a cheetah, the idea of a leopard never appealed to me. But I admired their lithe, muscular beauty even more than that of the lion.

Lulu was discovered by a ranger in the Eastern Transvaal region of South Africa, known as the bushveld; she was then very young, her eyes not yet open. She was taken into the ranger's home and reared on Lactogen; then, at the age of two months, she suddenly developed a fierceness which surprised even her foster-father, and started to show definite and aggressive signs of interest whenever she saw a dog or a small child. At this point Terry Reilly was asked to take her on; it was known that he was exceptionally skilled in the handling of wild animals. Without hesitation he undertook to rear the growing leopardess. Her aggressiveness was by now especially directed towards Africans; she snarled and flattened her ears at the sight of them, attacking whenever she could. This hatred of coloured skin was in no way related to any previous experience of cruel treatment suffered at their hands.

Terry and Lulu became devoted to each other in a very short time. They romped for hours, and from her new master Lulu would tolerate any amount of teasing, though coming from any-one else this would provoke unmistakable attack. Only once did she bite; Terry's mother was the victim, receiving deep wounds in her leg. This gentle and wonderful person knew and understood the ways of the wild as well as she understood her own wild son; she accepted the pain and discomfort smilingly and went about her farm, tending her animals and family without complaint as soon as she became mobile again.

Lulu was not a particularly intelligent feline; Terry often told of the many amusing moments when, chasing partridges up into the trees, she would leap off on to the ground below as soon as they flew off.

Now she was growing, perhaps more quickly than if she had been self-supporting in the wild. Terry usually kept her on a collar and chain when he took her among people; she had once disgraced herself by leaping towards the small baby of a friend with obvious intent to kill, but Terry caught her in mid-air and fortunately a disaster was averted. This made him aware of the danger involved in keeping her, even on a chain, and so he asked me to perform an ovaro-hysterectomy operation as soon as possible, thinking that this might quieten her increasing aggressiveness. She once slipped her collar and chain while Terry was driving home on leave to Swaziland and he did not discover that she was missing from her usual curled-up position on the back seat for some time. A tremendous search ensued but with no result. Terry spent a miserable leave, and two weeks later was leaving his farmland to return to duties on the Sabie Sand. Then, near some thick shubbery, within sight of a Swazi school teeming with small children, Terry thought he saw a flash of movement out of the corner of his eye. He stopped at once, though he had by this time given up hope of Lulu's survival. He mewed, imitating her cry; at once, as if catapulted, Lulu leapt into his arms, displaying overwhelming affection. Back home he drove, his heart singing. A feast fit for royalty was prepared for the now thin and mangy leopard, who had strangely resisted the temptation of killing one of the Swazi children. We have often wondered if she had managed to pick up her master's trail and simply dug in to wait for him, come what might, not even moving to assuage her hunger. Perhaps without him she lacked the initiative to kill or otherwise fend for herself; this is what Terry always assumed.

Some time later after this reunion Terry was sitting alone at his

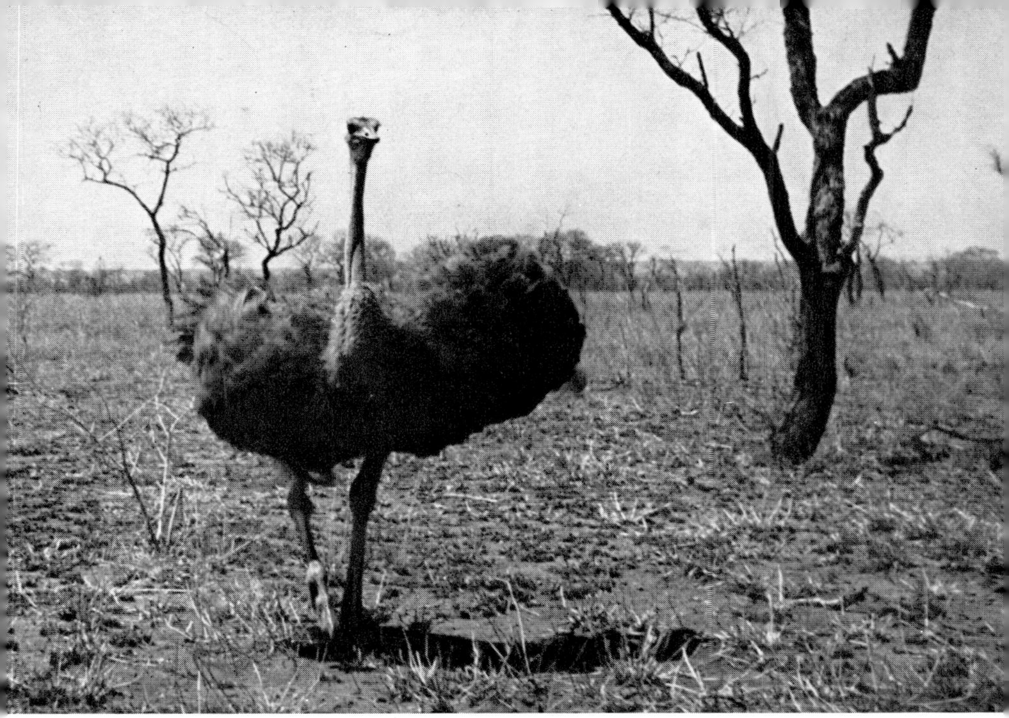

7. Twinkletoes, the ostrich enamoured of motorcars.
8. Lulu, the aggressive leopardess.

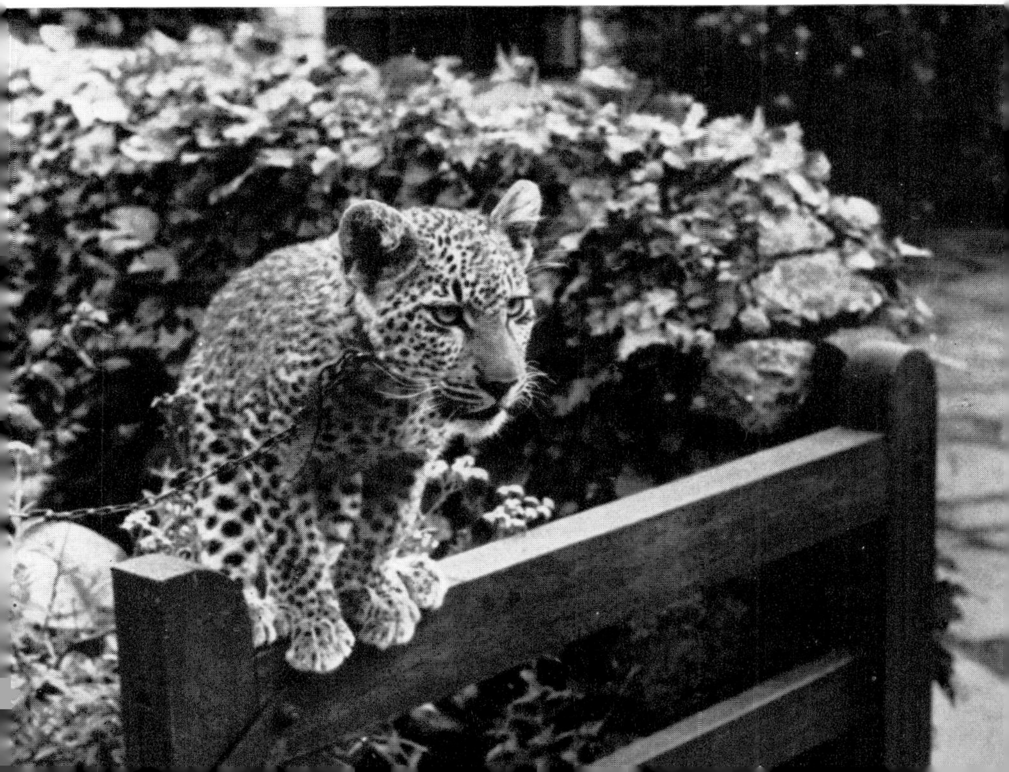

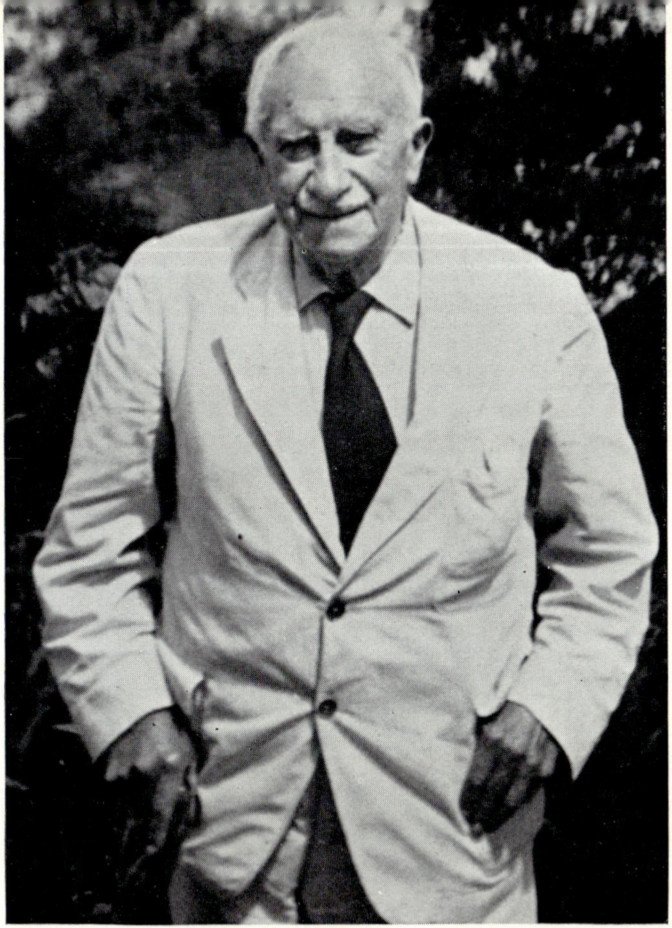

9. "Skukusa", who gave the world the Kruger National Park.

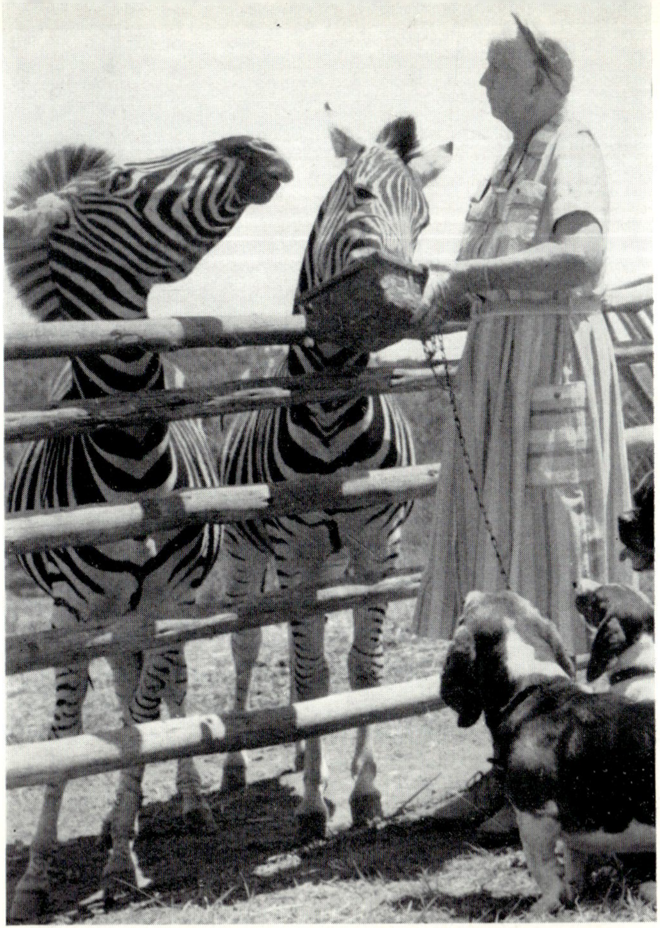

10. His wife, Hilda Stevenson-Hamilton, with her tame zebras and dogs.

evening meal (typical bachelor fare – mealie porridge, scrambled egg and meat; the first and only meal of the day), when he grew impatient; his repeated call to the cook had not been answered in the customary prompt manner. At last he went out to the kitchen, found nothing, and proceeded to the pantry: there a strange and ludicrous sight met his eyes. Lulu was crouched, ready to spring, snarling and menacing; the poor cook knelt, hands folded in supplication, repeating over and over again, as though in prayer: "Please don't eat me, Lulu; please don't you eat me, Lulu."

Simba, the bull-terrier cross, was her constant playmate and companion; this amazing dog had acquired some reputation as a formidable baboon killer. My very first contact with him had been to stitch his flank skin back on to his body, rather as one might darn a torn shirt which has been caught on a nail. He was a brave and heroic animal; his dislike for baboons arose from their habit of approaching the Land-Rover which he was guarding while Terry was off in the bush. Very few dogs live to tell the tale after an encounter with these ferocious apes; their strong pointed incisor teeth can rip a canine body from end to end, as they push it away with their arms after sinking their teeth into the flesh.

Terry Reilly's home was in Swaziland; his homestead lay at the end of a winding road that rose from the plains among tall pines and gums until the farm-house was reached. A tame impala or warthog was usually there to greet one even before the family appeared; looking across the valley of Mlilwane (named after the over-shadowing 'mountain of fire') one now sees the Game Sanctuary which Terry established in order to preserve and exhibit the wonderful wealth of wild life that Swaziland had, if man would only leave his heritage to live in peace. For political reasons the government withdrew the land which had already been allotted for a game sanctuary, and so he and his family gave their own farm of 11,000 acres and turned it into a game park. Here Terry brought zebra and antelope, giraffe, and white rhinoceros – this last not having been seen in those territories for a hundred and fifty years. It was a great triumph for him when, at last, Mlilwane Sanctuary was opened, and by no less a person than Hilda Stevenson-Hamilton, widow of the late warden of the Kruger National Park. Terry is an idealist; hardy, down-to-earth, devoted to the cause of wild-life conservation and protection; his knowledge is amazingly wide considering his youth. Against powerful opposition, financial difficulties, and the doubt of almost everyone who knew what he intended to achieve in that small area, he ploughed ahead, he built fences, he planned grazing and camp-sites, and he slowly won the support, until Swaziland could also boast of its own 'Noah's Ark'.

Apart from a few mountain leopard, the sanctuary contained no predators; zebra, giraffe, antelope, warthog, small buck and rhino as well as many species of beautiful birds can be seen on foot or from horse-back. The only danger which threatened when we visited the park was, of all bizarre things, an ostrich; one whom the children christened Twinkletoes because of his very fast gait. It was not completely clear whether he wanted our car or was just generally aggressive: but the fact remained that with one swipe of his ferocious toe he could inflict fatal injury. On one memorable afternoon he caught up with us while we were travelling in an open jeep, and in order to repel him we each threw at him the nearest object that came to hand. In my case this was the telephoto lens of my friend Howard Kirk, who had been foolish enough to entrust it to me; I aimed it at the chest of the threatening bird and managed to hit him square on the breast feathers. This repelled him for a moment, just long enough to give the driver time to bring the stalled engine into life; and after driving half a mile or so, we managed to shake off the bird, though he tried his best to slow us down by blowing up his neck, flapping his wings, and throwing his neck from side to side. When we were clear of him I suggested that we might return to retrieve the things we had thrown – the hats, sweaters, shirts, shoes and the telephoto lens. They must have been all together in a heap on the hard winter ground. I saw Howard change colour as he understood what I had done, but he sat immobile, mumbling something in shocked disbelief, his politeness preventing him from expressing his true thoughts. "But what could I do? All I had to throw was your lens, and I had to save the life of our friend on the bonnet! Would you not have done the same?" "No," came the chorus of many voices; and with some apprehension we began the search. Fortunately, only the diaphragm was damaged; and this Howard was able to mend for himself in the most expert manner. Recently, Twinkletoes has abandoned his habit of chasing people and cars,

ZEBRA IN THE MIST

and has taken his place in the family circle; he has proved himself a good father by helping to incubate no less than twenty ostrich eggs.

It was only during the winter months that I could afford to leave the practice for more than a few days at a time, for the large-animal work had dwindled considerably since the dry season had begun and ticks had become dormant at last. My practice then consisted chiefly of small-animal work, and on many occasions I longed to get out into the fields and forests, even to get stuck in the mud again, as so often before. I was consoled to some extent by my contacts with some of the most colourful personalities imaginable, living sometimes in the most inaccessible spots. Some of these were extraordinarily interesting, having pioneered the Lowveld in a past more remote than their faces or figures usually indicated. Many were experienced animal handlers and trainers, and I often dreamed of the days to come when through their inspiration more antelope and buck would grace our pastures, for their beauty and their utility value as well.

The only person who kept zebra was Hilda Stevenson-Hamilton, whose home overlooked the lake and some ranges of tree-covered hills that lay eight miles outside the village. If I were asked to choose my favourite place on earth, I would choose this paradise, wonderfully remote from the beaten trail. My family thought that my own farm-house home was in the wilderness, yet to me it seemed all too civilised, too easily get-at-able, too sophisticated altogether. In contrast, Hilda's Gibraltar – most suitably named after the rock formation on the lakeside – stood in an atmosphere of undisturbed peace. When in summer the valley below became a little too hot for comfort, it was glorious to escape to the ever-cooling breezes which softly stirred the leaves of the huge sentinel gums; quaint cottages stood in the unison and harmony of thatch, home-built of stone, grey as the grey wild rocks scattered among lawns and flowers. The extensive green sloped gently to the water's edge; to the left the eye was caught by a mass of Canna lilies flaming gold and red, planted on the edge of the jutting peninsula, below which bass rippled the water's surface at dusk.

Not far from here a pack of wild dogs had crossed on to the property shortly after Skukusa retired from his wardenship; the strange arrival of these wild animals, usually very shy of civilization, aroused much comment and speculation in the district, and the Africans were convinced that this was their mark of respect and farewell to the beloved chief whose labours had provided them with protection against man. The wild dogs disappeared even more strangely and suddenly than they had come, no one knowing whence they had come or where they went. The Colonel was greatly touched by the little episode, and perhaps his artistic soul strove to believe the folk-lore which this event initiated.

'Skukusa' means the man who changed everything: the name was given to him by members of the Shangaan tribe who were loyally bound to him, who respected and loved him for what he was, who worked with him and trusted him implicitly as one of themselves. This name will live to posterity; it is now more part of his tradition than the name to which he was born. Colonel James Stevenson-Hamilton, one of the greatest authorities on African wild life, became the first warden of the Kruger National Park, and remained there for forty-four years. He first came to South Africa in 1888 as an officer in the Sixth Dragoons and it was during his service in Natal that he first conceived the love of wild animals which later became the greatest interest in his life. In 1920 this great man undertook a venture and established himself in what is now the southern portion of this world-renowned National Park – renowned now, but completely unknown in the early 1920s. There, with little help and with only Henry Wolhuter as a fellow-ranger, with many misgivings, with enormous courage, assisted by a handful of African scouts, he planned and brought to fruition the development of this vast game sanctuary. The game at that time was very shy of the human form, because of hunters and poachers; and it took many years before these animals sensed that to stay was to live, to wander meant death.

The task which Skukusa undertook must have seemed overwhelming at the time; but he remained undaunted and fought his way to victory in the malaria-riddled bush country, where snakes and ticks and unknown diseases were plentiful. He succeeded so well that within only a few years the public began to support the Park. They arrived, mostly in oxwagons, to enjoy what the sanctuary had to offer; the experience was as new to the visitors as to the visited, and many a tale is still told in the Lowveld of unexpected encounters between human and wild animals, neither really prepared yet for the other's presence, neither aware that the days of aggression were ended. Gradually several camps were built, the first and foremost being in the south and named Skukusa; this became the centre of operations as well as the largest of all the camps. A beautiful library has now been built near the entrance of the camp in commemoration of the great pioneer; here one may browse or read at one's leisure in surroundings conducive to the study of the fauna and flora of Southern Africa; here the shelves are filled with every publication that a naturalist could desire. As one enters the library one is met by a life-size bronze figure of the Colonel himself, familiar fly-wisp in hand, so true a likeness that it is startling and touching at once. This is the creation of his devoted wife, who spent years modelling and remodelling it until it was perfect.

I first met Skukusa at a small luncheon given at an outlying farm, not far from his own home and still in sight of the lake. I had gate-crashed this party, for I was only there because I was working at Foresight that day. I had been called to attend a very sick old Jersey bull, special favourite of mine since he had the sweetest temperament of any Jersey bull in my experience: it is widely known how dangerous and unpredictable Jersey bulls usually are. This poor old veteran was suffering from Lumpy Skin disease, one of the most intractable virus infections: there is no specific treatment for it, but only symptomatic. Enormous plaques had formed and these were very extensive, covering most of one side of the chest wall, revealing necrotic flesh and deep fissures into the overlying muscle. The degenerating tissue had to be separated and removed as far as possible, an operation which lasted for hours, followed by cleansing and irrigation as well as general supportive therapy to improve his condition.

The bull, weighing about 1,500 lbs., offered no resistance, even latterly when his strength was returning; he simply lay there, turning his wise and powerful head backwards from time to time, regarding us with unmistakable understanding, only wincing or blowing slightly when the pain became too much. I had completed an hour's such work and returned to the homestead dishevelled, and no doubt emitting an aroma which is very difficult to lose at one scrubbing. The guests were about to sit down for lunch, and I was placed next to the Colonel: he engaged me in the liveliest conversation, asking me many questions about my work. My first impression of him was that of a man whose small build was counter-balanced by a dynamic personality. He had a kind, endearing smile and sparkling, humorous eyes, which nevertheless sized up everything and everyone around him with quick intensity. I was delighted to meet him at last; this had been a great ambition since I had read two of his books dealing with wild life in Africa. I had found these to be completely absorbing and full of detail, and I continued to use them as reference books for years afterwards.

And so I discovered what a fascinating person Skukusa was. Although he had retired, he still lived his work, and had in no way disassociated himself from it as many retired people do. He had started building up the Kruger Park late in life, for he already had a lengthy army career behind him. We talked about taming wild creatures especially the zebra; he had a dream of raising these on his estate, but this did not come true in his lifetime.

Skukusa died in 1958 at the age of ninety, one year after I had been privileged to meet him. We had formed a firm friendship and I hold most precious the memory of those hours spent with him and his wife, sitting on their terrace, speaking of the things that mattered most to us all. His books are the greatest authority on African wild life in the world. Yet in spite of the glory and fame which surrounded him, in spite of the homage which was paid to him from every part of the world, his humility and his modesty were a great wonder and a great lesson. His was a fine example of an ever-young mind; his happy philosophy and refreshing youthful personality were of the quality that could make the young feel old.

It was my habit to eat breakfast with them every Monday morning. We invariably sat in the open facing the lake, which was often still shrouded in mist, and enjoying the scents of the damp, new-cut grass, listened to the echoing song of the black-headed orioles as they repeated their challenging burbling call and moved from branch to branch. This was the scene of the morning of Skukusa's last birthday. We had managed to fulfil his wish to be given two kittens, ginger or Siamese, and he had received his present (Siamese) with evident and undisguised pleasure. He loved simple things, and as he lived, so he died; he gave an interview to the Broadcasting Association on the development of the Kruger Park, stressing his hope that the park would be kept as simple and natural as possible, and then he collapsed, and died not long afterwards. I was permitted to attend him during the last hours, and much of what he had achieved went through my mind as I sat with him. Perhaps there will never be another man who will leave such a powerful message to posterity; perhaps it is because of his unflagging spirit that the world is, at last, responding to the call of wild-life protection.

Some months after his passing, the zebras came to Gibraltar. I was myself responsible for the advent there of the first striped lady: on one of my early morning calls I almost collided with a black and white vision in the mist; I could not see too clearly, and I stopped, just in time to see an equine shape leap out of my path. When I arrived at my near-by destination, giving thanks for still possessing one whole and undamaged station-wagon, I inquired carefully, not wishing to create the impression that I was having hallucinations. I hinted that there might be a zebra foal roaming near by, and was rewarded by the farm-wife's confirmation. "There's nothing uncertain about that Duba. She belongs to our neighbours and she's a damn nuisance, always getting her head into the flour bin; tame in front, anything but tame behind!"

This really decided me; I had always wanted a little zebra, and I knew that Hilda Stevenson-Hamilton would be delighted to welcome one to her estate, even if only to train it for the initial period. Duba (the name is the Zulu for 'zebra') arrived on our farm shortly after my adventure at Hazy View, standing on the back of a huge truck, supported by two African labourers. As she approached the top of the drive we could hear the musical, almost whimsical neighing of the little foal; she was actually about eight months old, as her teeth and history showed, but she was not grown up nearly as fully as one in the wild would be at that age. The children were completely enraptured by her, and sad not to be able to keep her; but we deemed it wisest to transfer her to Gibraltar specially since her unpredictable back-kick could inflict serious damage to a child standing below four feet. She was put into the station-wagon, and we were soon on our way into the hills, headed for Duba's new home.

The little zebra settled down very quickly, chiefly because Hilda is possessed of the rare and wonderful gift of quickly winning the confidence of any animal. Within two weeks Duba was following her about everywhere, and although she enjoyed freedom, she was nevertheless given the necessary discipline to restrict her behaviour and make her a much safer companion. If something irked her, she first gave ample warning of her displeasure and took her time before kicking, thus giving a fair chance to those within range. Gentle and firm handling changed her from a delightful delinquent into an endearing friend; I delighted in having her around on my regular Monday morning breakfast visits. She would hover near by persistently, fluttering her unbelievably long eyelashes (lower lid only!) at us most lovingly, while all the while she ogled the fruit-basket at the centre of the table. I was never sure whether she was more attracted by the vivid green fruit-stand or by its contents; but, whichever it was, it became too much for her and she dived towards it unceremoniously, nose first, upsetting apples and oranges and bananas in every direction; she watched these with a look of satisfaction as they rolled down the sloping flowerbeds and between the roses. Often one or another of the dogs would get a direct hit on the nose from an orange, and this would be followed by a great show of howling to indicate that his dignity had been severely injured. All this would blend with Hilda's severe scolding; and the episode would often end in a dogfight between the jealous adolescent basset-hound, Brutus, and his unwilling companion, who could not see what there was to fight about. By this time, Duba, having discovered that her mistress's attention was distracted from her misdemeanour, felt reinstated; she would recapture the company's devotion by a skittish display of affection.

Some months later, when it became obvious that Duba was at last reaching maturity, a handsome stallion horse aptly named Star arrived as her consort, and became her constant and admiring follower, though regrettably never the father of zebra-cross foals. There was conjecture about this question for some months: Duba grew and grew in circumference during the rains, and even seemed to take on a matronly manner. Without wishing to disturb her by full-proof intensive inspection for pregnancy, I found the situation one of great interest; finally – though not all at once – the opinions of no less than four vets were sought to establish the truth or otherwise of her pregnant state. I was the last (and by far the least eminent) of the vets consulted; the whole episode gave me a feeling of complete inadequacy which, in spite of the humour of the situation, took a long time to live down.

Not only did we one and all decide that Duba was in a happy state of approaching motherhood; we went so far as to venture that her time was not far off. To make matters worse the head African, the faithful Strike, who had been with the family for years and had moved from the game park with them when Skukusa retired, firmly and unmovingly declared that it was a good season, and that Duba was simply full of nothing else but commonplace grass. We were shocked; we wondered how such a man, used to equines, could be so wrong, and so sure of himself at that! Hilda smiled, hoped we were right and thanked us all. In her heart of hearts she knew the truth, but was so hopeful and excited at the thought of producing a new kind of foal that she enjoyed conjecturing which part of the new-born would have stripes and which would be plain. We spent a few hopeful months this way, and, as happens only too often to those who count their chickens before they are hatched, we were doomed to disappointment. Yes, Strike – the ancient, stalwart Strike – proved to be right after all, for after some time Duba's girth lessened alarmingly and she regained her sylph-like figure in midwinter. Henceforth I held my horses before giving a rash diagnosis of pregnancy on the mare. Also, I decided never to trust too much in the opinion of other veterinarians, however experienced and renowned they were.

My weekly excursion to Gibraltar has been my weekly highlight for many years. If Monday was ever blue then this event certainly gave the beginning of the working week a rosy complexion. I usually aimed at leaving home by 6 a.m. on Mondays, by which time the children were up and dressed, my daughter practising the piano assiduously, while my little son, Guy, was busy feeding the guinea-pigs and pigeons and hindering Petrus with the milking. Life stirs early on those Lowveld mornings, for this time is the best of all and it is also the time when one's body-energy and one's mental concentration are at their maximum. The children caught the school bus at the corner of the farm a little after I left, and my own route took me to outlying but not too distant farms, where I could complete some work and still reach Hilda's home by eight o'clock. By the time I arrived I was ravenous, and ready indeed for the sumptuous breakfast which awaited me. Thus my working day was interrupted most pleasantly by this hour of relaxation and absolute joy, and this routine of the 'breakfast habit', as we came to call it, became very much part of my life.

Again and again I would stop and wonder and appreciate this wonderful life I led, one of hard work sprinkled with leisure and adorned by contact with people like Hilda, who lived every moment of the day with an intensity and creativeness which is surely the purpose of life. I pitied and sorrowed for those who never find their niche, either through a misunderstood or misdirected youth, or through that basic laziness which after a time becomes like a real disability. Perhaps it is the vast distances, the mighty forests, the mountains which give us humility, teaching us many things which we must understand in order to live more fully; and we can find much wisdom in the animal kingdom, and learn there the art of living close to the earth, and the sun.

CHAPTER 8

Famous People and Jungle Addicts

Most of us have certain and definite ideals in life – abstract hopes that we wish to fulfil, goals towards which we strive, personalities that we try to emulate.

For me, Hilda Stevenson-Hamilton is such a person: she is the most amazing woman I have ever met. The thought of her brings her back to my mind's eye as I so often saw her, standing in the slight shadow of the covered walk, next to the uncannily life-like figure of Jock, a previously owned and much-loved dog, whose image she had herself sculptured after his death. I see her, arms slightly raised in a welcoming gesture, her clay-covered working apron still on her, smiling as only she knew how in a fashion at once shy and deeply heart-warming, her staccato voice bursting across to me over the pink and white roses: "Hello, dear Sue" nothing more or less in words, but always much more in meaning. To see and hear her thus was to me, each time, a new homecoming.

She is a person who lives close to the earth and the sun, reflecting the sun's energy which she daily pours into her creative artistry, living in close kinship with the earthiness of the animal kingdom. Much younger than her celebrated late husband, she is, at sixty-three years of age, ceaselessly active. To telephone her after six-thirty in the morning is useless, for by that time, whatever the weather, she is up and about on the farm, organising the African labourers, working with the host of garden boys, inspecting the black oxen that are still used for pulling water-drums from the dam in time of drought, walking over the fields with the dogs, training the zebras, going about endless tasks which entail the covering of much ground, uphill and downhill.

When I arrive at about eight o'clock in the morning, Hilda has already achieved half a day's work while most 'lords of the manor', specially the local type, are just staggering out of bed, unable to focus without the aid of a strong cup of coffee, or even a glass of whisky. She is a joy to be with, for her agile mind and impish sense of fun are tremendously stimulating. Sometimes she has quite exhausted me and put me to shame by cheerfully suggesting that before breakfast we should do a tour of the pigs and then leading on, with long strides, to the dongas (deeply-graded slopes and holes) through bramble and fern into the shrub, to locate the pigs. She kept them for love, and they responded to her call by appearing immediately from all directions in large numbers. By this time I was usually covered in thorns, my stomach rumbling with hunger; even the thought of returning to the homestead, through the bushy slopes and declines, made me go weak at the knees. Then, when we were almost within sight of the breakfast table, Hilda would suggest that I should sex her geese before we eat, since she was expecting guests that luncheon and wished to slaughter one of the male birds in good time.

The first time I was asked to perform this task, I had little clue about how to do it; it was something that had escaped me in my college course, or (I suspect) something that had not been taught to us at all. I muddled through as best I could, finally achieving some sort of efficiency and certainty as to how to establish the sex of birds, hoping that if I made a mistake this would never be detected from the taste of the roast. Each time I sexed a goose, a band, appropriately red or blue, was firmly placed on its leg, so that I would not be needed on future occasions. In actual fact this did not work out, for the geese cleverly managed to lose the bands, and so each time I came, which was frequently, I sexed the whole flock all over again.

Finally, having completed the sexing amidst much flutter of feathers and farmyard chaos and confusion, we settled down to a hand-scrub which had to be lengthy to be any use at all. After that breakfast was heaven; it took all my self-control to restrain myself from eating the last four pieces of toast, which were always reserved for the dogs – a routine upon which the new and unwary visitor was soon enlightened. Hilda loved getting all the local news from me on this weekly visit, for she seldom went out anywhere, preferring to have her friends come to her. My work reached every part of the community and she revelled in the anecdotes and news-flashes that I presented to her on these occasions, often listening to some amusing tale with tears streaming down her face.

She is, above all, an artist, and one well-renowned for her vivid and life-like animal drawings which have been and are still widely used as curtain designs in the Kruger National Park. Everything she depicts is vibrantly alive: the antelope seem to be gracefully and delicately moving across the cloth, the lion and leopard are ready to spring upon their prey. Her elephants tower with lofty dignity above the warthogs, which seem to be ever rushing and running somewhere, in family line, tails held stiffly up. These forest inhabitants not only have the true-to-life shape and movement, but they are possessed also of a subtle grace which comes from the infinite love which Hilda has put into her drawing.

I have, on many occasions, stayed at Gibraltar; there I seek peace and solitude, there I can write, think and live without disturbance. I have, on occasion, gone there to recover from illness, and have been treated with such loving care that my recovery has been startlingly rapid. And who would not revive in such a haven, where the air is scented with the fragrance of roses and honeysuckle? – one or other of which Hilda has always, most thoughtfully, placed in her guest-room. There is a rare and absolute stillness which one can actually hear, not disturbed by the sound of dogs barking, or by Banjo's (the boxer) regular patrol of the domain, his opening and closing of the screen doors at his every coming. The engine, the chattering of the guinea-fowl, the reed brooms on the paths in front of the windows – these sounds merely melt into the stillness.

The four dogs form the most unusual ensemble, as diverse in character and behaviour-pattern as in shape. Banjo, whose nobility is evident at once (his real name is Beau Geste of Ruwenzori), is the most stable, most loyal and most reliable; he protects Hilda from intruders, tracks down the chicken-thieves (a task for which she has trained him), and is in general the leader of the band. Then, next in seniority, comes Walkyrie, an ancient wrinkled bloodhound cross, like a prehistoric shape dressed in an oversize skin. Her sight is failing but her nose is still good; so is her bay, which, heard at night, reminds one of beheaded ghosts and medieval castles. Brutus, the bellicose basset-hound, has an aggressive and unpredictable nature; he is happy to pick a fight at a moment's notice, especially when he knows that no one really takes him seriously. Last comes Siam, a young beagle bitch, who is feminine and alluring in the extreme. Hilda, who is a strict disciplinarian, rules this bizarre foursome with stern and gentle kindness, ready to punish or to praise, with absolute justice – a treatment that she extends also to the many servants who adore her and serve her with gladness. When her head man gets drunk, Hilda handcuffs him and immobilises him until he is sober, a treatment to which he has no objection at all, since it obviously protects him from the actions which all drunks are apt to inflict upon themselves and others.

I have been fortunate in being invited, with other friends, to visit the Kruger National Park with her. The private camp at Skukusa, originally designed and built by her when her husband was warden of the Park, is pleasantly fenced off from the remaining huts and public area; the little enclosure always has an air of peace and privacy, even when the main camp is teeming with hundreds of visitors. To visit the Reserve with someone so much a part of it is a truly wonderful experience, for here she is on very familiar ground and knows every tree, every hyena burrow. I have heard some amazing stories from retired Park rangers, depicting her life in the wild. Coming across a lioness one day, while she was walking through the bush on foot to find good sketching subjects, she reacted to the situation exactly in the opposite way to what one would expect. Instead of giving way or beating a hasty retreat when faced with the aggressive beast, she simply continued on, looked the lioness in the eye, and called "shoo, shoo" in the same sharp, commanding voice that one uses for children, or cats. It is said that the lioness, perhaps sensing a complete lack of fear, gave way in an instant and trotted off obediently.

On this particular visit we drove to Orpen Dam, about ninety minutes to the north. This is one of the few beauty spots where one is permitted to leave the car and observe and watch in the open for as long as one likes. Standing so high, one gets an impression of looking down on a sunken stage, a stage of tremendous activity, most of it invisible to the beholder, even with binoculars. One overlooks a rocky, aloe-filled decline; to the right lies a *koppie* (rocky cluster) where leopard live, ready to pounce upon the unsuspecting thirsty antelope. During the previous year, when the lower road could still be approached by the public, I witnessed the attack of one of these leopards upon a drinking waterbuck male. Such sights are usually unpleasant, but this was rather an amusing episode: the leopard was obviously still very young, without very much experience in the art of catching his prey. He rushed in full view, towards the antelope, his advance clumsy and slow and cub-like. By the time he reached the spot, his quarry had disappeared into the forested slopes; but the leopard was not able to check his attack, and almost landed in the water. I shall always remember the comical expression on his face, which seemed to say "Well, I'm damned, I could have sworn there was a waterbuck here, only a moment ago!"

Looking down across the water, we could see the hills very clearly, thinly covered with acacia trees. Peering into the distance, we gradually detected the dark shapes slowly filtering down to the water, arriving, as it seemed, from nowhere, in ones and twos, collecting into a widening stream, as they approached and converged at the water's edge. It was past eleven in the morning, the sun's rays giving a slow but sure increase of heat, the signal for those in the wilderness and forests to quench their thirst.

A huge crocodile had made its home in the Orpen Dam, and whenever I have been there I have detected it lurking in the depths where it waits, like the leopard, for a chance to satisfy its hunger. On this day of our visit we detected it from above, seeing only the eye-ridges, even these being barely visible above the water. Waterbuck, kudu and impala, eager to quench their thirst, nevertheless refrained from drinking, sensing the danger without actually seeing it. Witnessing this drama was as tense and exciting as any film I have ever seen; although the outcome, we realised, might be a death and an unpleasant one at that, we were too fascinated to move our eyes from the scene for a single instant. We searched the surface for tell-tale ripples; the crocodile had suddenly disappeared from sight, and even from above we could not detect it for a time. The impala, the least wary of these beasts, now came down to drink; slowly and surely, with delicate tread, they reached the muddy edge. For a moment we were deceived that the crocodile had really left and the throb of heartbeat lessened in our ears. Then suddenly, just as the thirsty ones stood bent to drink, quick as a flash the black shape was there among them, heaving itself out of the murky current, snapping its jaws so violently that the vicious sound echoed across the valley like a gun-shot.

Though Nature's laws must not be disturbed, we could not help feeling a thrill of joy and relief when the little buck escaped.

The rest leapt back and galloped up the slope, coming to a halt some distance away; here they stood in surprising calm, waiting for another chance to drink. Before long, and perhaps because their memories are short, they slowly and hesitantly filtered down, this time venturing much farther, wading down the muddy bank. We wondered if this drama would now repeat itself, and again we waited with bated breath, while the photographer in our party, hoping to get a unique sequence, sat glued to his camera, his telephoto lens trained upon the scene. We should have allowed ourselves to be guided by the more certain and less fearful behaviour of the impala, for the crocodile had really departed this time; no doubt everyone present, except us, was aware of this.

On another occasion the impala did not get off so lightly. We had just passed one of the rock-pools of the Sabie river when Howard, whose eyes and ears are sharply aware of the most distant event, suddenly braked and reversed, saying that he had heard something most unusual. We sat and listened for some moments, tuning into the bird-filled world which is silent to those inside a motor-car; and gradually we became aware of sporadic crunching and snapping sounds beyond the trees in the river. At the same moment we spied a mass of flailing jaws and flashing fangs, the body of the turmoil moving closer to the shore at each moment. No less than seven crocodiles were consuming what must have been a very large impala, some ripping at the partly macerated body while another attempted to dislodge a limb-segment from its lower jaw. This crocodile disappeared under the water at intervals, apparently finding it easier to deal with below than on the surface; slowly it managed to move the obstruction, until at last the whole piece had disappeared down its huge gullet.

The thrashing and gnashing of teeth finally abated, after we had watched the scene for over half an hour. We wondered if, at such a reptilian feast, there was any order of division of the carcase, any equal apportionment, such as there often is in the wild. It is interesting too to know that crocodiles, one of the most

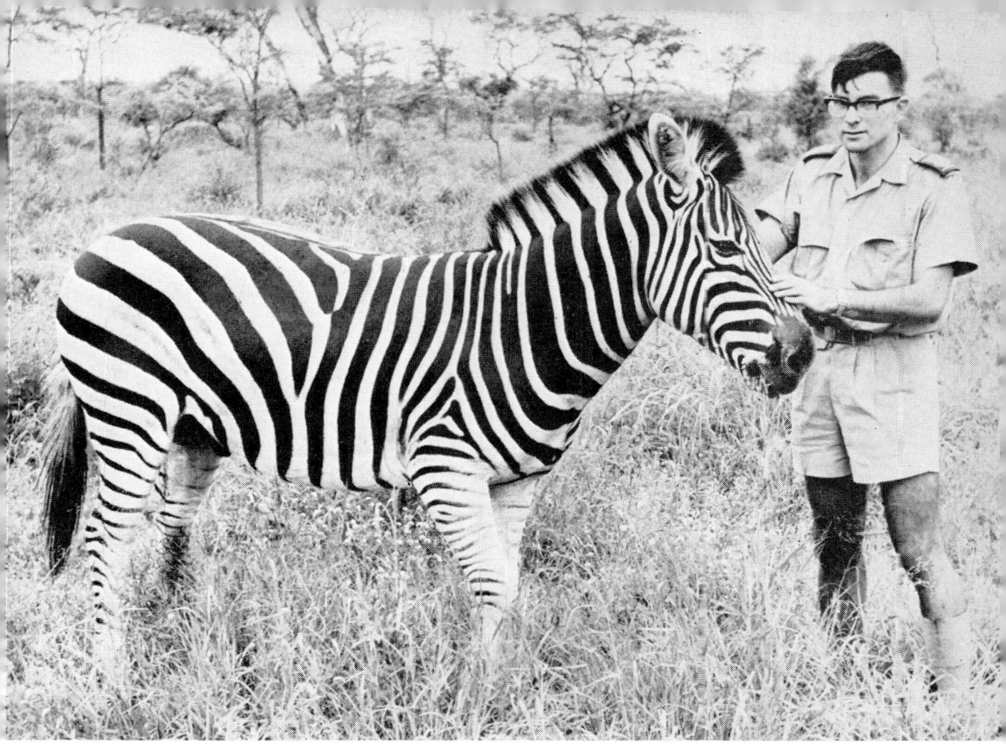

11. A wild zebra standing quietly after immobilisation with M99.
12. Scientists carrying out physiological research on an immobilised elephant.

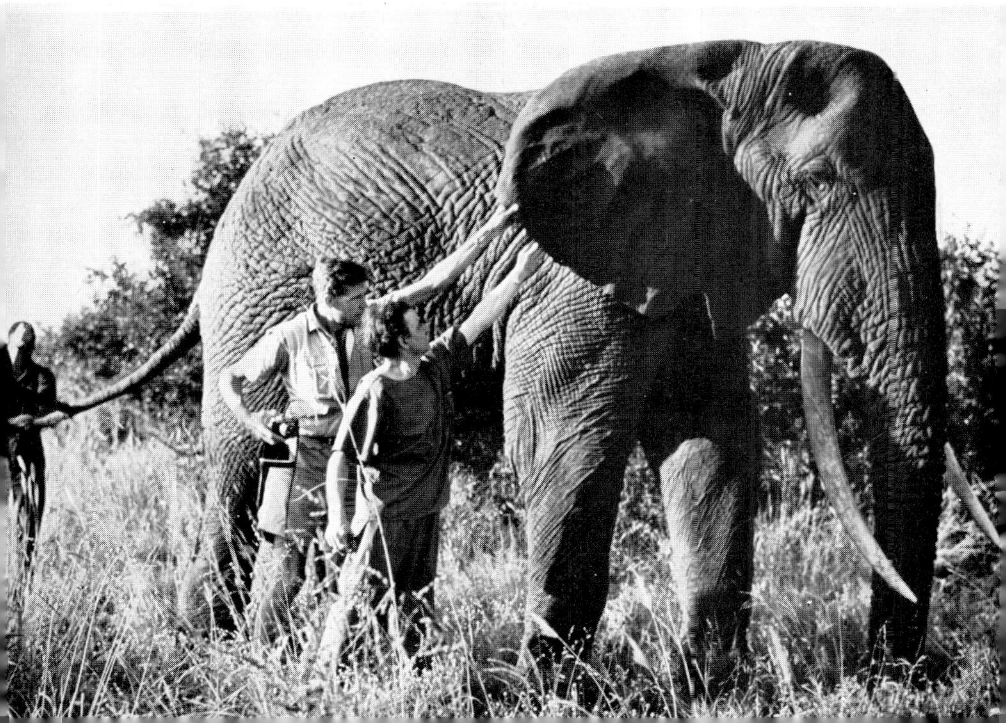

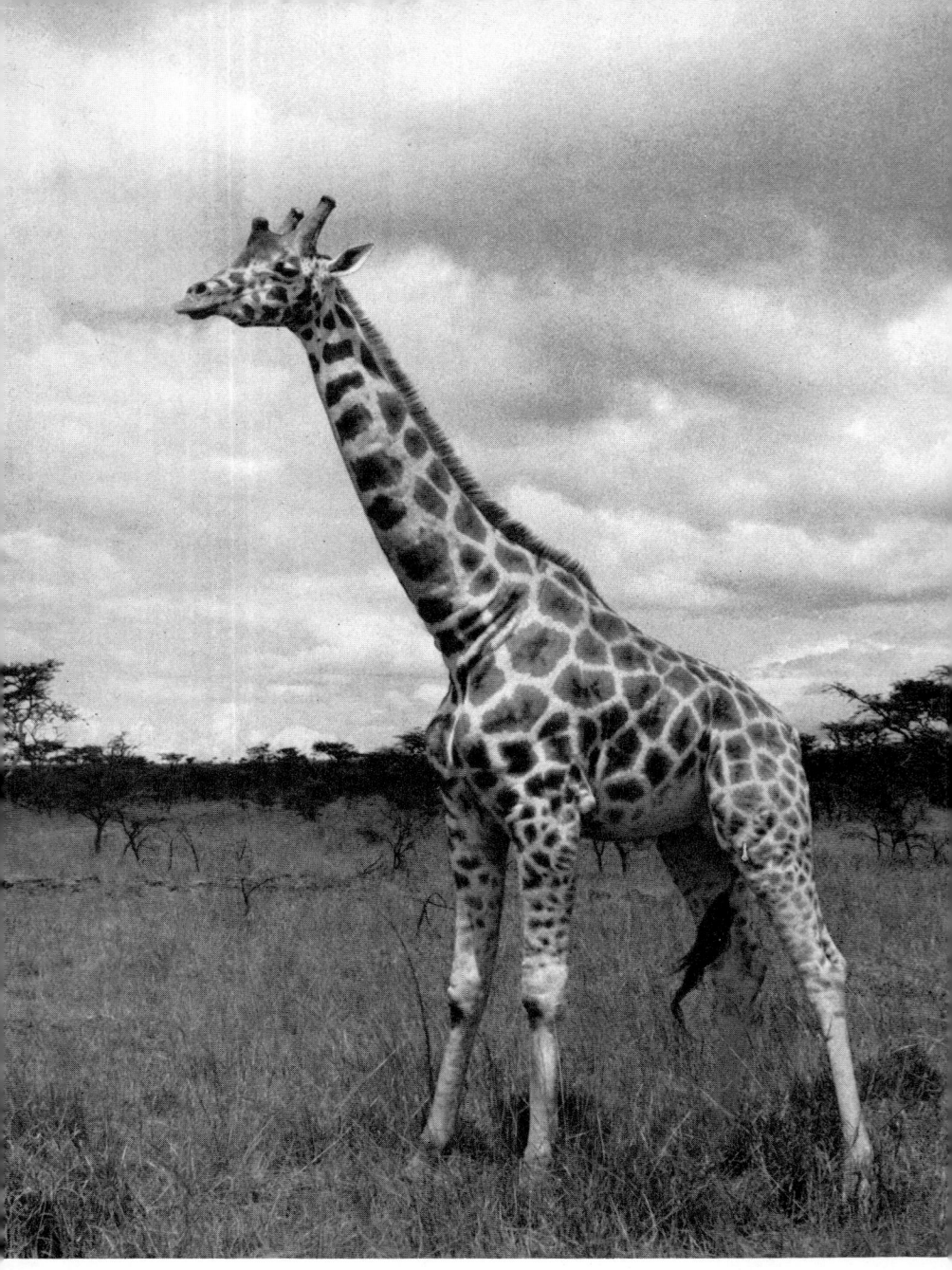

13. An immobilised giraffe. Note the dart still attached to the hind leg.

misunderstood of wild animals, are not greedy, wasteful and aggressive carnivores as is often believed; true, they will take an unwary buck when the opportunity arises, but they usually live on predatory fish, such as the lung-fish, which in its turn feeds largely upon the valuable fishes which man enjoys. And so the crocodile fulfils a useful and not a villainous role.

Although we were gazing straight in front of us, we did not see the elephant until he came quite close. Like a grey ghost he emerged from the shadows, plodding silently along the well-trodden game track, looking neither right nor left. As he neared the drinking antelope, he shook his great head and ears, displaying his impatience at their trivial presence. "Out of the way, small fry!" The small fry took the hint and retreated a little, making room for him, being obviously used to the bluff of the good-natured giant. An exquisitely marked male giraffe, standing in apparently deep thought just to the left of the elephant's path, did not give way as did the antelope and buck. Two warthogs, also ignoring the massive threatening intruder, were drinking from a shallow puddle, minute against the background of long, dappled legs.

I had perched myself on top of the rocky slope, leaning against a camphor-tree, catching every sound which drifted from below and above into the midday haziness so characteristic of Africa. Two hippopotami, old residents of the dam and well known to us all, honked good-naturedly at intervals, the sound travelling back and forth across the water like a fog-horn. In startling contrast came the high-pitched call of the orange-breasted shrike; the green spotted dove, perched near by, burst forth again into its mournful Morse-code song: "to- totoo- tototoo- tototoo- to- to- to- to- to- totototoo". . . . The Zulus, steeped in folk-lore, have interpreted this sad song as meaning "they have killed my father, they have killed my mother, they have killed my children, and my heart goes to- to- to-. . . ."

The elephant, having drunk his fill, now began to splash and blow with gusto; when he tired of this, he lay down against the muddy bank, half submerged, like a dog seeking the coolth of a puddle. By this time we had sought the shade of the recently erected reed shelter, while the kudu and waterbuck sought the protection of a large and spreading maroela-tree, patiently waiting for the elephant to leave so they could claim their water-rights. At last the mud-caked king arose, causing tremendous commotion among the antelope as he made his dignified exit towards the east, a striking contrast to the restless, fairy-like impala, their soft brown merging into the background, their presence only revealed to a casual glance by the momentary flick of their white tail underfluff.

Two purple-crested louries came into view, their startingly red-purple wings making me blink; in the distance the regal fish-eagle circled his domain, the valley capturing his haunting unforgettable call. White egrets, temporarily leaving the antelope-hosts upon whose ticks they feed, settled on the banks of the dam, watching the furry waterbuck drink their fill. All about me, yellow and white butterflies wove their strange pattern of jerky flight, disappearing below the rocks that merged into the carpet-like masses of dense yellow flowering water-plants. A ruby-red dragonfly hovered to my left, then came to rest upon a dry stick beside me, leaving it again after a moment to hunt for flies; I watched it for some time, as it returned time and again to that vantage point, vibrating, its head down, its wings exquisitely fashioned and translucent. A yellow-billed hornbill, the most extroverted comic actor of the bushveld, perched on my camphor-tree, dramatising some tale of the bush with his bubbly, uninhibited song. For a brief moment a pair of brown-hooded kingfishers glided alongside, leaving almost immediately to find some more restful and private perch. Three African lily-trotters glided along the nearest strip of water-plants, their huge webbed feet giving them tremendous speed. A grey-and-black barred harrier-hawk swooped down from the heights, to seek for prey but finding nothing, then left us far behind with a few beats of his powerful wings. The quiet of this beauty-filled scene was broken by the puffing and blowing of the hippos; reluctantly we rose to leave, knowing that most of the wonders of that place had not been revealed to our limited senses.

Like any other ordinary visitor, I had always been confined to the tourist tracks and roads, though I yearned to go off into the bush and to move freely, away from the crowd. The opportunity to do this came quite unexpectedly; I had done nothing to deserve it, but I had the good fortune to have as friend the distinguished

FAMOUS PEOPLE AND JUNGLE ADDICTS

physiologist and veterinary scientist, Dr. A. M. Harthoorn of the University of East Africa. Now he was invited to come to the Kruger National Park to demonstrate the use of a chemical substance he had developed for the immobilisation of wild animals. I was already acquainted with the scientific staff at Skukusa, because I lived near to the park and had my veterinary practice adjacent to its area. Now I became one of them, part of the team which set out to do this amazing and most interesting work. The controlled movement of wild animals was first attempted in 1958 at Lugari, Uganda, when thirty kob antelope, a rare Kenya species in grave danger of extinction, were moved in order to establish a nucleus of this species in the Mara triangle. This area, lying on the border between southern Kenya and Tanganyika (now Tanzania) was then a protected area and is now listed as a game reserve. About that time giraffe were also transported, from farmlands at Nabiswa on the edge of the Karamoja in northern Uganda, to the Menengai crater near Nakuru, Kenya, which was protected and safe. At this time immobilising methods were still in their infancy, and experience was being rapidly gained in this field as the need arose all over the world for transporting wild animals.

It was in 1959 that Toni Harthoorn went to Kariba in Southern Rhodesia to attempt the rescue of the black rhinoceros which were in danger of their lives as the area became flooded. These rhino had to be removed as quickly as possible. Other game had been caught, more easily, by the efficient teams headed by Rupert Fothergill, of the famed 'Operation Noah'; but the rhino had refused to leave the islands to which they had retreated and, unlike other animals, they showed mistrust and fear of water. It was up to the scientists to find a way to move them, if possible, without injury. Toni Harthoorn had for some time been experimenting with certain substances which had the effect of quietening animals so that handling and movement would cause little or no alarm; the recovery from these drugs would be gradual. He came to Kariba with the purpose of attempting to move these animals with the aid of such drugs; they were injected into a muscle mass using barbed darts, fired from either capture-guns or cross-bows. This method proved successful, and many rhinoceros were moved to new and safe land.

At this juncture, the substances which I saw used in the Kruger Park had not yet been evolved, or even thought of. This came later, in 1960, when Colonel Vincent – then Director of the Natal Parks, Fish and Preservation Board – invited Toni Harthoorn to come to Zululand, so that over a hundred white rhinoceros could be moved in order to ensure their survival. These events, which revolutionised wild-life conservation and gave hope for the continuance of many threatened species, aroused wide interest. For the first time in history, wild animals could be studied at close quarters without destruction, and fact upon fact was revealed about the amazing life-patterns and physiology of the African mammals. Public conscience was deeply stirred, and it seemed as if man and animal would be brought, none too soon, into closer and more meaningful relationship.

Toni was a physiologist, and his interest naturally lay in the study of the normal functions of the animal body. The advent of immobilising drugs opened up a new field of discovery; now, at last, study could be made under almost normal conditions, and the animals could afterwards return to the wild. Through his work in this field, science acquired a new dimension; although burdened with academic and administrative responsibilities, he worked at this hobby (as he called it) until he had found a substance so safe and successful, that the world of animal preservationists acclaimed him as the man who saved wild life in Africa, the Albert Schweitzer of the animal world.

When Toni Harthoorn came to work in the Kruger Park, he brought with him a chemical substance, known only by its serial number as M99, which was a synthesised morphia-like compound a thousand times more powerful than morphine. What looked like a few grains of salt was, in fact, strong enough to immobilise twenty elephants; and it had this additional and vital advantage, that it had an antidote – its effect could be reversed by an antagonistic solution, with immediate effect if this was given intravenously.

The scientific staff of the Park had already done some work in this direction, and certain animals had been moved under the influence of other drugs. Now they wished to familiarise themselves with M99 which was already used by the Natal Parks, as Toni Harthoorn had spent some time there previously. For two weeks a team of scientists, veterinarians and other helpers including students, went full out to perfect the new method. I myself arrived one week after the work had begun, almost missing my rendezvous because an enchanting family of cheetahs displayed itself distractingly on the route to Skukusa, and almost made me forget why I was there. Cheetah are unfortunately very rare indeed, and to see a whole family of young with their mother is a great stroke of luck. There was also a young adult male present who was intent on marking out their territory: he did this by rapidly climbing a roadside tree and marking it with urine, doing this several times on different branches, and with great concentration. I doubt whether I would have understood this procedure, had I not seen it once before when in the company of a naturalist, who explained this type of territorial or land-ownership behaviour-pattern to me. It is widely known among ornithologists that birds mark their territory by simply showing their presence and singing along their borders: a much more refined way of asserting ownership!

I entered the Skukusa administration offices at 10 a.m., and was immediately whipped away to a waiting Land-Rover which transported us to the field of action. It was possible to see the tracks of other vehicles before us, and the exact place where these had turned off the main road (never tarred) into the bush. Our first indication that we had found the working location was the sight of a darted kudu cow; the team was following her up, but we spotted her first. She was wandering along, rather unsteadily, circling an area of thick bush. She had been darted some eight minutes before, and the drug's effect was approaching its maximum. Her fear of man was gradually disappearing, and her natural timidness and tendency to avoid strange sights and sounds was changing into the opposite: she approached the Land-Rover without apprehension, only shying away at the last moment. The rest of the team were now at hand, quietly watching, ropes ready, observing and timing the antelope's moment-to-moment actions. Toni Harthoorn was there, tall and lean, watching and controlling the operation with his usual calm and concentration, commanding respectful attention to his every word, since he always spoke with measured knowledge that comes from wide experience. There he stood, stethoscope round his neck, testing equipment tucked into his specially made-to-measure bush waistcoat, recording sheets in his hand; a man with the unusual quality, which so many scientists lack, of being able to combine his thirst for knowledge with a love and consideration for those from whom this knowledge is gathered. He handled animals with care and consideration, and ensured that everyone involved in the work did the same.

It was not long before the kudu slowed down completely and stood leaning against a thorn tree, quite unperturbed now by the surrounding activity. In contrast to previously used compounds, when immobilised with M99, an animal does not fall down, but remains standing, which is much safer for it.

At this juncture, I was invited to leave the vehicle and to watch and help with the procedure. The kudu was caught, roped, and marked with a coloured collar for future observation; then records of temperature, heart-rate and respiration were made, and body measurements taken. This only lasted a few minutes; the antidote had meanwhile been made ready and was now administered into the jugular vein, this being raised by application of pointed pressure anterior to the shoulder blade. The effect was instantaneous: the ropes had already been detached, and the animal leapt to its feet and galloped off without looking right or left, anxious to leave us behind as fast as possible, its natural fear and suspicion flooding back in one instant.

Having never witnessed immobilisation before, I was utterly astonished by this first experience of it. It was so incredible that it was some time before I could absorb it and begin to understand the implications. That a completely wild animal should become amenable and manageable in such a short space of time; that it should then, in a flick of an eye, revert to its previous state without undue harm and probably with no memory of what had occurred; that it should allow itself to be approached a second time, if necessary: all this seemed to me nothing short of a miracle. But this was only the beginning; I knew nothing that morning of future and yet more remarkable developments, but I did appreciate my own good fortune in being allowed to be part of this experience. I was, perhaps, the first woman veterinarian to be allowed to work in the wild anywhere.

The next few days were very lucky ones: I was told that if luck is out, hour upon hour can be wasted in searching for the elusive quarry. We seemed to find, almost at once, the exact animal we were looking for; and so within a short period of time many species of game were immobilised – giraffe, elephant, zebra, wildebeest, waterbuck, tsessebe, impala and many others. The range of the cross-bow, which the Park's scientists were using at the time, was up to eighty yards; this means that careful driving, good manoeuvring, accurate estimation of animal body-weight, and excellent marksmanship were required. When the country was open, to follow up darted game proved relatively easy; but in bushy, uneven terrain, such as we encountered when following up a herd of magnificent sable antelope, it was extremely difficult to get an uninterrupted view and to take undisturbed aim, and the darts sometimes bounced off from intervening twigs and branches. Very rarely did an opportunity present itself a second time, and many hours were often wasted before a good shot could be made.

The marksman engaged on this work has to aim very precisely, usually at well-muscled buttocks or shoulder. Sometimes the projectile-syringe strikes too gently and only penetrates the subcuticular and less vascular tissues (those tissues lying under the skin which contain only a limited blood supply); the drug is then absorbed much more slowly. Then the dart-mechanism may fail, or the dart may drop out or be brushed away before much of the liquid has been injected: again, the projectionist cannot be sure how much of the mixture has entered the animal's body. It is known that certain of the antelope, such as the impala, actually deflect the dart with their horns; their reaction-time is so short that they register the whizzing movement of the projectile, take instant action, and turn the missile aside – in a fraction of time barely perceptible to the onlooker.

Elephant in the Kruger National Park have very little antipathy or suspicion towards man. They react when aroused or teased, they often amuse themselves by playing road-blocking tricks on tourists, they pull down 'Beware of Elephant' signs with regular monotony; but otherwise are friendly and unconcerned when viewed from a distance and treated with respect. On one occasion a mishap occurred because some motorists, though seeing that elephant wished to cross to the river, nevertheless blocked the path, with the result that one of the cars lost its streamlined shape and the driver and passengers were severely shocked. They demanded that the miscreant be destroyed at once, presuming to pass judgement in a situation which they could have avoided. The authorities, with absolute justice and heartwarming and unprecedented firmness, issued a statement declaring that the Park was a sanctuary for wild animals; the public were invited to visit it, providing they conformed to the rules. We who took the animals' side breathed a sigh of relief; the new attitude so expressed showed a swing in Park policy. In future, people would take second place to animals. This gave us a gleam of hope in our battle against hunting and poaching.

Toni Harthoorn was always surprised at the amiability of the Transvaal elephant; in East Africa, things were different. On one hot afternoon, we spotted a huge bull peacefully browsing among the acacia trees. The sound of our engines did not disturb him in the least, and the dart was fired under optimum conditions. He hardly reacted to the impact of penetration, only showing a slight irritation by ceasing to feed and beginning to walk, pacing slowly while we followed at a respectable distance. After twenty minutes he stopped, swayed a little as though leaning against an imaginary tree, continuing his slow walk after a few moments, but this time in circles, ever narrowing. The drug-mixture was obviously taking effect, and we quietly waited for the moment when we could approach more closely. He was estimated to weigh about 12,000 lbs., with 80 lbs. of ivory on each side; such lovely tusks would have been the sure cause of his destruction had he not lived in protected land. At last he halted about one mile from the spot where we had first found him, and simply stood, drunkenly unsteady, while we approached, keeping well out of reach of the trunk which was still fairly active. He was aware of us, but did not seem to worry about our presence unduly while in the drugged state.

To me he seemed simply enormous; there was something majestic and awe-inspiring about the grey-wrinkled king of beasts. Although by man he had, for a time, been subdued, man, standing in his magnificent shade, seemed insignificant. His huge ears still maintained their rhythm, moving regularly back and forth: this movement has recently been shown to be the elephant's radiator or body-cooling system.

The usual method of reversing the drug action was impossible in this case, for the ear-veins could not be reached, except by means of a step-ladder, which no one had remembered to bring. The antidote was therefore injected intramuscularly, taking effect very quickly in this case – so quickly, in fact, that we had to retreat to our respective vehicles as fast as we could. Another elephant which went down with the immobilising drug was somewhat easier to measure and monitor, and I was given the honour of taking his rectal temperature. I was, at first, at a loss how to achieve this task; I ended up lying flat on my stomach, heaving his tail into the air with my left hand, and plunging in with my other, hoping that I was doing it all correctly. The others laughed, but had no advice to give: no one had ever taken the rectal (or any other) temperature of any elephant in the wild state before. I was amazed and delighted to find that the temperature of this and subsequent elephants was similar to that of the human, i.e. approximately 97 degrees Fahrenheit – assuming, of course, that the immobilising compound had little effect on the internal thermostatic control system. Perhaps this is our one and only point of similarity with these majestic beasts; if so, so much the worse for us. From that time on I was appointed recorder of internal temperatures, a post not entirely unfraught with danger: the rangers and scientists made a practice of administering the antidote, with immediate and startling effect, while I was still hanging on to the tail.

The giraffe, so unlike his jungle brothers in every way, also responded distinctively when tranquillised with M99. He behaved consistently and without variation, and the team worked out a plan of action which was successful in almost every case. Apart from the usual slowing-down reaction, the giraffe, after some minutes, demonstrated a typical arched-back posture, coupled with a turned-upwards-and-backwards head-position and a stiff high-stepping gait, hardly if at all noticeable in some of the antelope. On the whole these bizarre animals were not perturbed by our presence; some of the game scouts would walk alongside armed with ropes, waiting for the moment to extend these across the animal's path. If the right moment was chosen, the giraffe would simply stop as soon as his movement became restricted.

On one occasion, however, even a phlegmatic, easy-going

long-neck became disturbed. This was due to the irrepressible enthusiasm of a learned Professor of Biology, whose greatest interest lay in the study of animal symmetry and particularly of the skin markings of wild animals. Unable to restrain himself, this elderly gentleman, in shorts and top hat, leapt across the path of an enormous slowing-down giraffe, and dived under his belly before he could be prevented; then he had to keep pace with the animal as it accelerated dangerously, sensing that something very unusual was beneath its undercarriage. He was visible now on this side and now on the other, always somehow avoiding the deadly hoofs. We were frozen to the spot, astonished and very alarmed; the biologist in charge, a kindly man, lost his self-control, and muttered strong words – a reaction completely warranted, since only one hour earlier the same professor had got himself lost in the steaming trackless forest and had not even expressed gratitude for his eventual rescue.

The giraffe had, most unfortunately, been disturbed out of his dreamy state by this time; this was possible, since morphine-like substances create a state which can be broken if the animal is agitated. Sometimes, if quiet ensues, he may become calm once more, but this time the animal had been startled too thoroughly for this. The professor, covered in thorns and perspiration, miraculously escaped without harm; then the team had to devise a way of catching the giraffe before he went out of sight. It was not safe to let him get away without antidote in case he fell prey to predators, yet to re-immobilise him was not completely safe either, since no one could guess how much of the substance he yet retained, and a second dose may have been too much. It was therefore decided to head him off and allow him to become entangled in the ropes. This procedure took some time; the photographers, laden down with equipment, in the burning sun, had to move fast and far to keep within photographic range.

While the giraffe was down, he vocalised most emphatically, emitting a bleating type of sound which is rarely heard; fortunately one of the party had a tape-recorder with him and was able to record this unique sound for all time. Much has been written about the 'silent' giraffe, even to the extent of describing him as the only animal without vocal chords; I myself had never heard his voice before, and I was a little disappointed that instead of producing a call as unusual as his appearance, he only uttered a most ovine, and not very musical sound.

The rest of this episode proved to be uneventful, which was just as well, since we were all quite worn out by this time. The giraffe, true to type, rose as soon as the antidote was injected, and cantered off into the thicket, glancing at us somewhat disdainfully (in true giraffe fashion) as he went by.

Like most people I had read widely about this type of work; and imagined myself to understand it thoroughly, especially since I lived so near the Park. When I had spent a few days as part of the immobilising team I discovered how wrong I had been; only now was I discovering what was actually involved, and I would go on learning about it for the rest of my days, though at the time I did not know how closely I was to be linked with this work. Whenever human beings discard their normal anxiety and avarice and give their strength – and often their health as well – in the service of the animal kingdom, another small step is taken towards a positive and hopeful world in which man may, one day, be able to hold up his head without shame. It is tragic that progress is so slow and that so very few are bearing upon their shoulders the enormous burden of work which is the responsibility of so many. These few – not more than a handful of men – have given their days to the cause of wild-life protection, and to the study of how this can best be achieved. In Zululand, Natal, one species has been saved; the team which achieved this worked night and day, suffering much hardship and even injury. The world heard about them, admired them, and then forgot the whole subject, not seeing that this was only a beginning. The re-location of species whose existence is threatened is something so new and so fantastic that it should be shouted from the rooftops; now at last, by the methods of humane tranquillisation and immobilisation, needless suffering and loss of life can be avoided.

This work is truly a labour of love; the rangers who devote themselves to it, their faces unknown and their pay shamefully inadequate, live lonely lives, often enforcing unavoidable loneliness upon their families too. To see and share and live with these valiant few, even for a little while, is an extraordinary and very humbling experience. They are absolutely selfless and completely devoted, and they get tremendous joy from what they are doing. I shall never forget the end of one most tiring day in the Kruger Park, when the team – exhausted from the intense heat, covered in dust, parched for lack of water – was on its last lap home to camp. Suddenly an infant warthog went scuttling into the side, almost touching the wheels as it disappeared. Acutely aware of every smallest happening, the driver stopped, and as one man the carload leapt into the bush to catch the errant baby. I was surprised at this episode, and could not understand the cause for all the fuss, especially as I was badly in need of home-comforts myself at the time. But when the struggling baby pig – a charming little individual in spite of the unappetising nomenclature of its species – was safely trussed and secured, it was explained to me that a warthog family never divides, and that the mother always keeps close to her young in any circumstance – any, that is, except death. To the rangers it was clear in an instant that this warthog piglet would be devoured by a predator unless taken to safety and reared, since its mother had obviously been killed – not too long before, judging by its good condition.

This little incident showed me once again how kind and soft-hearted are these men who work with the wild. Strangely enough, they are often people who have once had the hunting-lust and who first had to get this urge out of their system before they turned from destruction to protection. It also demonstrated, once more, how much I still had to learn about the bush and the forest and their inhabitants: I had to admit to myself, reluctantly, that my bush-ears and bush-eyes were still more than half-closed.

CHAPTER 9

Songololo in my Bed

Beauty is a very subjective thing, seen and cherished by one where another sees nothing. So it was with my sister and I. Her face would light up with joy at the sight of a blotched canvas entitled Restless Sky or Rocks Adrift, or some other such name, while I would shudder at what the artist had dared to identify with a natural scene. We shared a love for music and for laughter, and had similar tastes in many things; yet as soon as those rocks had left the canvas and become part of raw nature, her need for pavements, high walls and street lights immediately reasserted itself. She loved the buzz of cities, the cocktail crowds, the streamlined homes whose electricity and plumbing functioned with uninterrupted efficiency. She rejected my love for the wild as vehemently as I rejected life in the cities.

Nevertheless she braved the wilds about three times a year to visit me. I felt that my farm was far too tame; she did not share that opinion, and she stayed with us only for the shortest possible time before fleeing back to the concrete jungle. Her two children loved my kind of life in spite of their city upbringing; her vivacious daughter Jacqueline, in particular, was a true chip off her aunt's side of the block. My poor sister Alice, having had to contend with a younger tom-boyish sister throughout childhood, was once again faced with the same sort of personality: Jackie loved riding horses, milking cows, examining strange *gogas* (insects), and pulling grimaces of the kind that used to send her mother into hysterics when we were children.

Alice, herself an artist, loved to use bird motifs for the creation of her lovely batiks, yet was unwilling to spend much time out of doors, where those very same birds could be observed in their natural surroundings. For us, visits to the Kruger National Park were a delight; for her, they were agonies which somehow always ended in disaster – nor did she ever really see any game. She went from a sense of duty, for the children's sake and perhaps she chose unlucky days; whenever she arrived back home, hot, tired and disconsolate, she swore that she would never again enter the Park as long as she lived. "What can you possibly see in it?" she would ask, "cooped up in a steaming car all day, endlessly shaken to bits at a speed of 25 m.p.h. – that isn't my idea of fun! If we only had the diversion of occasionally seeing something it wouldn't be so bad, but I never see anything except a few brown buck, and they are all identical anyway."

What amazed her was that so many people indulged in this brand of lunacy, often wasting their meagre savings and their annual holidays on this self-inflicted torture. Being always unlucky, she found it hard to believe that anyone ever saw anything. It was her own antipathy that kept the animals away; or so her little son, Ian, suggested. When Alice returned to Pretoria and was besieged by friends who wanted to know how she had enjoyed her visit, her retort was honest, though it surprised them: "Next time I want to see wild animals I'll go to the zoo; it's much less trouble and far cheaper. That Kruger Park is grossly overrated; you're choked by the dust of other cars, and when you need a few moments' break for one reason or another, you aren't even allowed to get out, except in a few far-between places. People who are otherwise quite balanced and normal seem to become quite daft once they cross into the Reserve; they will stop you, though you are a complete stranger, and ask if you have seen a lion. If you say no, they won't let you go until they have told you in detail where they saw one for half a minute three hours ago. If you say you have, they won't let you continue until you have explained in even greater detail where you saw it. I tell you, if you want to preserve your sanity, don't take one step towards that terrible place!"

During one winter, there was an unusual quantity of game in the southern areas of the park; an unprecedented drought had forced most of the antelope, smaller buck, zebra and wildebeest to come for water along a stretch of the Sabie river that is easily watched by visitors. Lions were plentiful that year; this gathering of their prey made them concentrate along this stretch for many months, and kills were often seen. Elephant, cheetah and leopard had been spotted as well as the carnivorous camp-followers, the hyena and the jackal. I was determined that Alice should somehow be persuaded to brave the Park once more; I was sure that this time she could not fail to revise her opinion. I asked my friend, Howard Kirk, to take her and the children in for a few days, knowing him to be not only a wonderful guide but also a great authority on birds and beasts; a journey with him would be an unforgettable experience.

They set off full of hope to Pretorius Kop, the most southern gate, laden with enough food to last them for a month. I congratulated myself on this plan and enjoyed the next days more than usual, wondering several times each day what my sister's family might, at that particular moment, be seeing. Perhaps a tawny-spotted cheetah pair, with rough-coated cubs; perhaps a pride of magnificent lions, stalking their prey along the river banks; or perhaps a leopard, feasting upon a kill which it had dragged up a tree.

I had booked the party in for only three days and four nights, but fully expected them to stay for much longer; I knew well that once the mood of that magic bushveld captures one, it is almost impossible to tear oneself away. Great was my surprise, therefore, when on the third morning the car drove up and out tumbled my family, looking hot and disgruntled, their guide haggard and pale, a far sadder man than the one I knew. What could have happened, I wondered with anxiety; surely he would not have taken it so to heart, even if there had been a sudden scarcity of game. They stumbled into the house, begged for tea and only began to relate their tale of woe after the hot, sweet fluid had revived their spirits.

It appeared that poor Howard, at a cocktail party the night before they set off, had eaten some sea-food which must have been in the process of deterioration. About the time they reached their first night camp, he had collapsed with nausea and dysentery, unable to go a step farther. His illness had lasted for two days, during which my sister had ministered to him as best she could and the children had amused themselves in the camp-ground. On the third day, when Howard felt a little better but still far too weak to drive, they decided to call it a day and admit defeat. "It is just fate," Alice sighed with resignation, "I am just not meant to go into the Wild. This finally proves it." And so I had to agree reluctantly that perhaps she was right; and thereafter I planned no more trips into the bushveld for her.

It was a strange coincidence that whenever she and her children came down to the Lowveld, either our smooth-rhythmed water pump, or else our electric light which had not failed since its installation, or else our one and only lavatory, would refuse to function. We were used to such incidents, and found candles and lamps no harder to accept than a dearth of fresh water or a faulty cistern. I had always preferred soft lighting and regretted the day when the harsh bright lights had been installed with no real advantage other than a piece of toast in the morning. Once I announced to the family that I would try to get out of my legal contract with the electricity organisation, before the installation was completed, and I was amazed at their violent reaction. "We won't come and visit you any more; we can't stand living in this almost-darkness, when you cannot even see if you're stepping on a snake!" This line of thought forced me to install the lights after all: had I hesitated any longer, it would have looked as if I wanted to keep the family away!

Later on, when we moved into a bigger farm-house which boasted two bathrooms, my sister and her family rejoiced, promising to make more frequent visits to enjoy such luxury. My sister now had the use of a superb *stoep* (covered veranda) on which she could spread out her things and paint, with a view of the surrounding mountains spreading in every direction. The new house was completely gauzed in, thus ensuring that creepy-crawly things would stay outside; though sometimes this security measure broke down, especially when the numerous dogs we kept learnt how to open the gauze doors, without learning how to shut them. "It's a palace," my sister would say joyously, "how to live in the wilds of Africa and still be civilised!"

But she spoke too soon. At this time my practice was expanding considerably, and I took an increasing number of ambulatory patients into the house, since many of my clients came from far afield and could not consult me very easily about aftercare. I sometimes housed as many as twelve patients at a time, ranging from canines and felines to monkeys and injured wild buck. The overflow from the outdoor kennels, and all the most serious cases, were looked after indoors. I decided to allot one of the

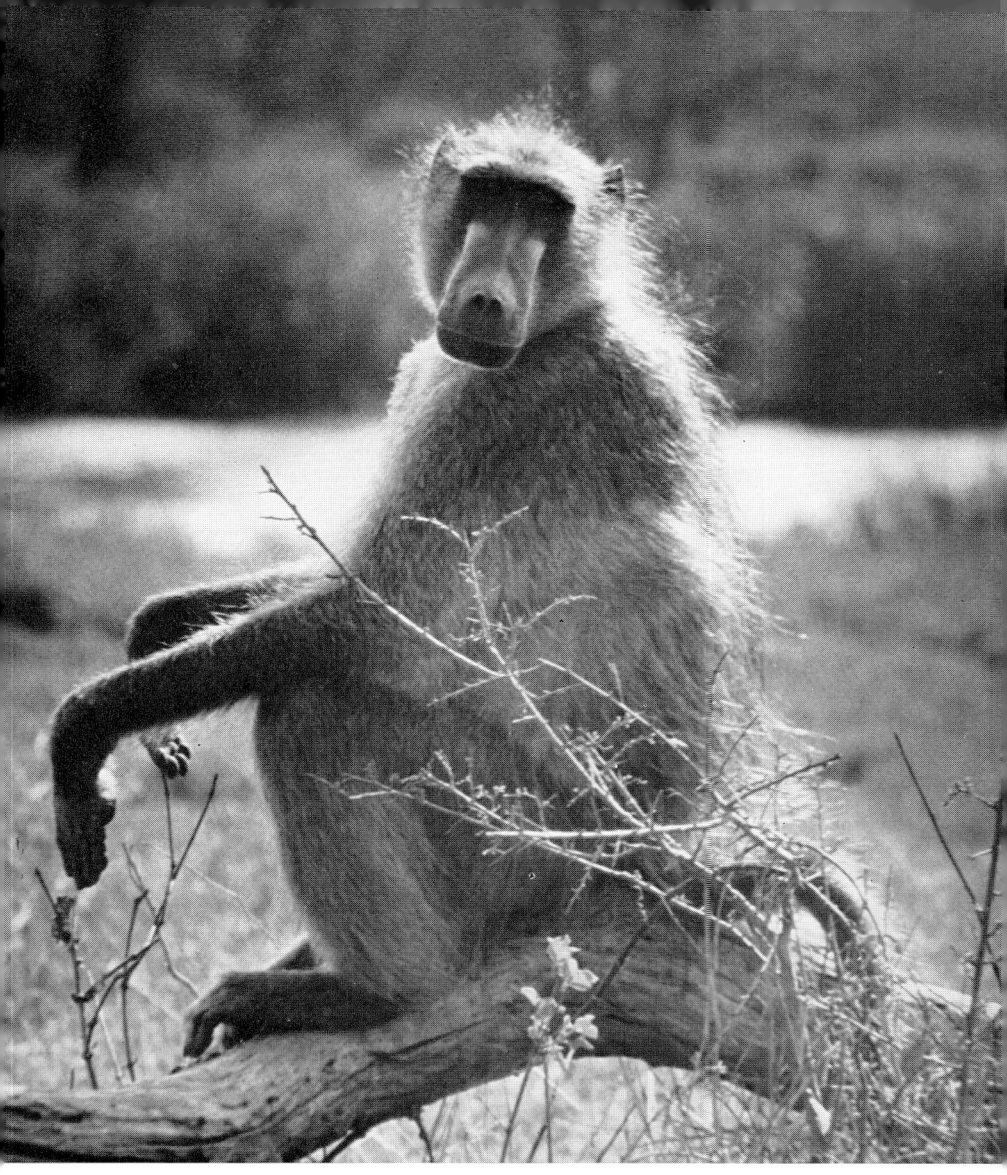

14. A baboon. These animals can inflict terrible injuries.

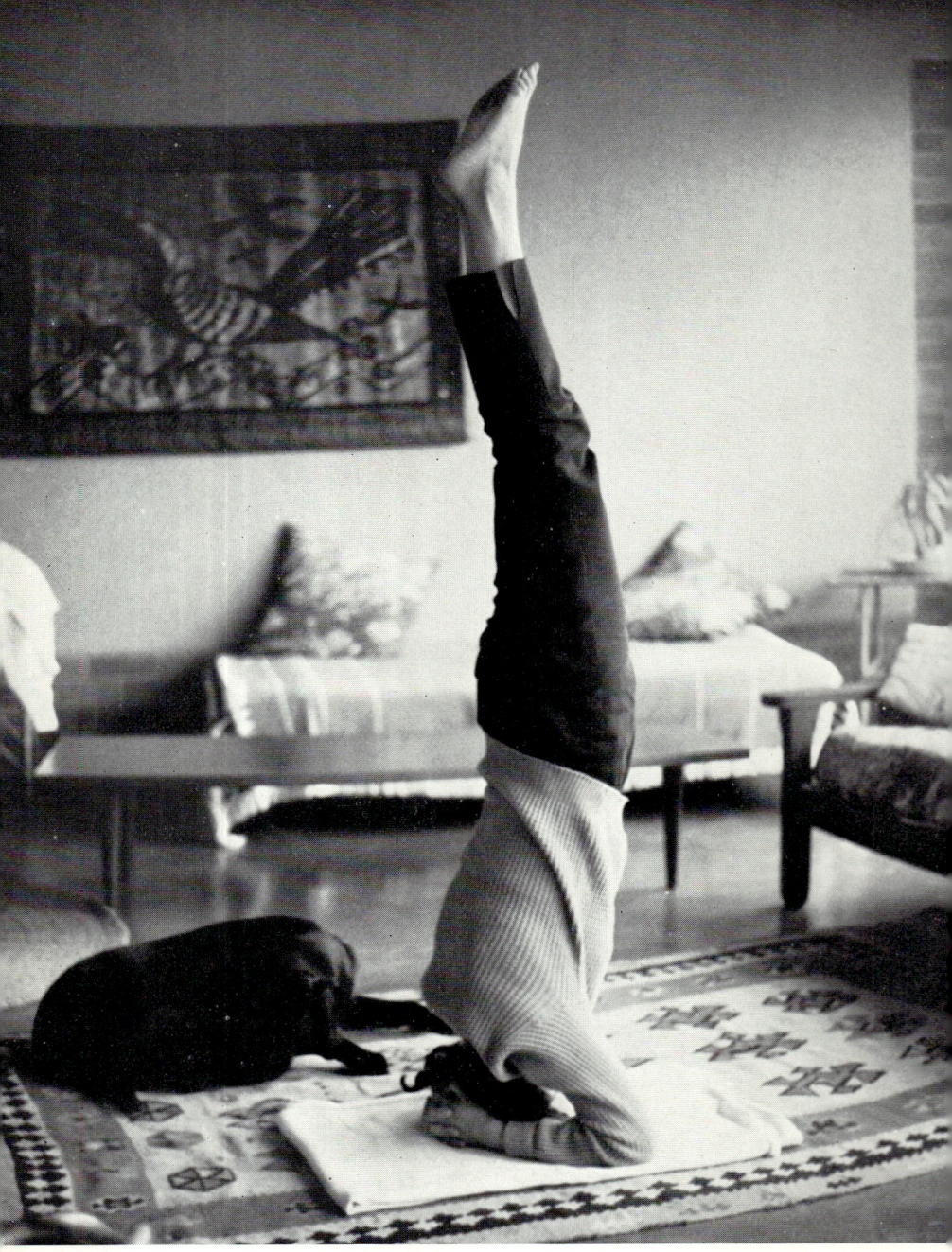
15. Everyone, including the dog, was used to this Yoga exercise.

bathrooms to children and guests, and kept my own bathroom – which had the additional comfort of an interconnecting dressing-room-cum-study – for myself, my most needy patients, and my sister, who always shared that end of the house with me. Sometimes, when emergencies arose, the other bathroom (which was tiled and easily cleaned) became a hospital ward; and this became a routine measure, to such an extent that the children, after a weekend away, would ask, immediately on returning and before opening any door, "Any sick animals in the bathroom, Mummy?" If I replied in the affirmative they knew at once that the opening and closing of doors had to be fast and silent: the patients' needs came first. To my own little family and those of my friends who stayed with me, this became an accepted situation. But for my sister, whose house was adapted strictly for human occupation, it was an ordeal to have to climb over a recent amputation case, with odorous dressings and sensitive temperament; it seemed to spoil the pleasure of her bath, even if I had taken the trouble to deodorise the room with powerful pine tar bath-oil.

There was always something new and exciting (nerve-racking, she called it) going on; and in the end I admired her immensely for her heroism in the face of such adversity. On one memorable occasion she offered to cook the dinner; I was very busy with late-afternoon cases, and she always had a horror of my doing anything in the kitchen in the interval between treating some ghastly disease and attending to a calving cow. She insisted – perhaps rightly – that the results and remains of such labours could not be erased in one scrubbing, and that it wasn't fair to expose the food of one's guests or family to contact with such things. And so she planned a wonderful meal, just to please me and my wild farmer friends, as she called them; and exploring the deep-freeze compartment of the frigidaire in search of some frozen steaks which she had bought, she unwrapped one of the tin-foil packages and found, instead, a very sizable and recognisable portion of a dog's head and brains which I had forgotten to warn her about. I entered the kitchen at that moment, and saw her turn white as a sheet; I was just in time to save her from total collapse. Gradually she recovered from this shock and bravely promised to continue what she had begun, although I knew full well what agony she was undergoing. Very unwisely, as I was leaving the kitchen to continue my work, I explained to her just why the deep-freeze compartment had been so very useful to me: she had unwrapped the brain of a dog which I suspected of having rabies, and this could only be sent on to the veterinary research institution after the weekend. This was the end of her courage, and I cursed myself for not keeping quiet: I was forced to cook the dinner myself, but I greatly enjoyed the version of the story with which she regaled our guests over the dinner-table.

To one such party, a rather larger one, I invited some of the local Italians, excellent musicians and entertainers; and my pride was hurt deeply, for I discovered on this night that I was dispensable, even in my own home. Just as the guests were beginning to enter into the spirit of the dancing and singing under the leadership of a gifted Italian carpenter, I received an urgent call to attend a cow in calving difficulties. I changed my high heels for rubber boots, removed my ear-rings and bracelet, covered my star-spangled dress with a white overall, whispered explanations to my sister and my cook, grabbed my medical case and other paraphernalia and drove off into the night.

I felt guilty at leaving my own party, and hoped that the proceedings would not suffer from my absence. I guessed that by now everyone knew that I had been called out, and felt some sympathy for me; and I imagined that until my return things might not go too well. When I arrived at the farm, I found, to my intense relief, that the considerate cow had managed to deliver her calf without my ministrations: all that was left to do was to check her internally and see that all was well. The farm was only ten miles away, and within one hour I was back home, none the worse for wear except that I needed a thorough scrub to erase the evidence from my arms. I entered the house as quietly as I could; I need not have bothered, for the joyous sounds of soft music and animated voices drowned all other noises anyway. It seemed that this gathering was self-sufficient and needed little help or encouragement from its hostess! I redecorated myself as quickly as I could, threw the dirty boots into the back garden, examined my dress for any stains, and returned to the large veranda, full of anticipation.

As I entered, a ginger-haired aggressive young man, whom I had never seen before, came up to me with a welcoming gesture and invited me to dance. "And who might you be, beauteous signorita?" he asked happily, "you are just in time for the fun. Isn't this a wonderful party, quite extraordinary, considering that our hostess is a he-woman with cow-dung in her hair who throws bulls and does terrible things to male dogs. I haven't met her yet, but frankly, between ourselves, I don't really want to meet her. I don't like amazons and bearded women; now you're the sort of girl I could go for in a big way, what do you say?"

Fortunately for me, at that moment, the crowd was asked for absolute silence while the Italian tenor furniture-maker gave a heart-moving rendering of the famous aria in 'Rigoletto'. This saved me from being forced to answer my partner's last question, and I managed to slip away from him during the uproarious applause which followed, to lick my wounds and attend to the serving of supper. How to stay away from this offensive young man for the rest of the evening: that was the problem. I would have succeeded but for my conscience-stricken friends who, upon taking leave in the small hours of the morning, sought me out from among the egg-and-bacon-and-coffee battalion in the kitchen. "Terrible not to have introduced you before, Sue; this is our friend Ginger Gape, who has been staying with us; he's training for the Diplomatic Corps. We felt sure you would not mind if we brought him along." "I am afraid you may have to change your choice of career," I could not help saying, limply, and to the surprise of my friends. "Delighted to have had you at my party." Ginger Gape's expression was hazy as he retreated from view. "Good night, enchantress," he muttered, "I have a feeling we shall never meet again."

Most civilised people love to lie in after such a late night: this would certainly be considered normal in a normal household. In my own establishment, however, which few would consider strictly normal, my house-guests were rarely allowed the luxury of peace and quiet next morning. Dinky, our charming grandmother-donkey, would come at six o'clock to bray lovingly at our window, wanting nothing more than the handful of sugar which, on weekdays, was always given her at the surgery window. Her call was something very special; it may have stemmed from the fact that like our cow, Lucky grew up in the company of dogs, her early vocalisations being somewhat confused as a result. Her first notes were long, low and drawn out, something like an old-fashioned car trying to change gear on a steep hill; gradually they took on a higher pitch, and just as the listener supposed that she had finished saying what she wanted to say, she would break into a bray of such intensity as to suggest numerous donkeys on every side. The black father-donkey (named Tinker Dot by the children for some reason I have never discovered) was totally blind, and had been saved from being slaughtered as hyena-bait for an ardent photographer; at this point he would begin to answer Dinky's call, even though it was not directed at him at all. He was usually at the end of the orchard in the very early morning, standing head to tail with his daughter, Longears, of whom he was inordinately fond. The braying of the trio, though it would gladden the heart of any donkey, drove my slumbering sister to despair. Though she had lived and worked and slept through the noise of enemy bombs and shattering glass during the long war years in London, she could not retain her equanimity when three asses exploded outside our windows: and she would shoot out of bed as though a bucket of iciest water had been emptied over her. "Can't you control those damn monstrosities?" she exploded on one occasion, "they would waken the dead. Why don't you cut their throats?"

One morning her grumblings and cursings fell on my empty bed: I had risen at the early Sunday hour of eight o'clock and gone out to see an injured duiker, a small buck which had been tormented by dogs and brought down by them after a lengthy chase; the owner of the dogs, a kindly farmer whose gentleness contrasted oddly with his huge bulk and his powerful voice, had interfered with the hunt and saved the life of this beautiful fawn, for the time being at least.

Alice rose from her last tortured moments of bray-filled sleep, and struggled over my latest post-operative case to reach the bath; just then, Sam the cook knocked on the door, announcing the arrival of a neighbour and friend. He had come to discuss something very important and was happy to unburden himself to my second-in-command, since I had already left. Sam was a very intelligent person whose work included cooking, assisting at operations, handling and nursing, gardening and any other jobs that happened to be going on at the time; he also had the uncanny gift of knowing everything that was going on in the neighbourhood, but he was diplomatic enough to keep most of this knowledge to himself – knowledge which he no doubt acquired by bush telegraph, the fastest news-service in the world, travelling as the crow flies, either by drum or whatever other unknown means.

My sister had no wish to discuss anything with our neighbour, probably thinking that he had a message concerning some animal which needed treatment; but Sam was insistent, and waited in the passage until she emerged so that he could perform the necessary introductions. "This, Doctor's sister," he said, as he backed out, "and this, our neighbour." He returned some moments later, smilingly bearing a tray of coffee, after which he discreetly withdrew and closed the door.

I learnt on my return what had happened during this clandestine interview. Alice met me in the passage as I opened the front door, her face contorted with worry, and before I could ask what was the matter, she drew me into the lounge and closed the doors.

"Your neighbour has been here," she began.

"I see that," I observed, "he has left another packet of beautiful oranges for us."

"Never mind about the oranges," she cut in impatiently, "he came about something quite different."

I felt hazy and tired all of a sudden, for the effect of red wine and lack of sleep, combined with a tiredness which resulted from grappling with the little duiker's wounds, left me exhausted and limp. There was only one certain and immediate cure for this, and I had to apply it immediately if anything sensible were to come out of the next ten minutes. "Forgive me if I conduct our conversation upside down," I said, "I feel I need some extra blood in my brain."

Whereupon I took an old blanket out of the mending basket, placed it next to my dog Cheetah, and got on to my head. Everyone, including the dog, was used to this exercise; and I think that in her distraught state Alice barely noticed that alteration in my posture. (She enjoyed doing Hatha-Yoga exercises as much as I did.) However, to spare me the awkwardness of having to speak upside down, she sat in silence for a few moments, until I felt sufficiently refreshed to get off my head and sit down next to her.

"Well, is his ram sick? – perhaps I should not have taken him off the antibiotics so soon," I said eventually. "Does he want me to go over?"

"Now, listen!" said Alice tensely, "What I have to tell you is *in no way* connected with oranges or rams. He came to tell me about the *lions!*"

My heart sank with dismay; I knew that hunters were in the vicinity, and had hoped that this news would not reach the house. "Please don't worry about them," I reassured her, "I had heard some story about lions wandering out of the Park for lack of food, but they are bound to be far away, in the bushy valley."

"Do you mean to sit there and tell me that all this time you *knew*? You knew the lions were hungry, and yet you let the children move about as usual, visiting their friends across the way? Really, this is *too* much; I shall just have to take them home, before something terrible happens."

Alice was really at the end of her tether, and I am afraid I was not being very helpful. "They are far away and just as afraid of us as we are of them, you know. Forget about our neighbour, and let's go out for a picnic."

"Your neighbour has just told me that only this morning lions' hair was found on his fence-strands, and that we should not go too far on foot."

This rather startled me, and I was just thinking how to cope with this new situation when the children burst in gaily, shrieking in their excitement, stumbling over the chairs in their competitive efforts to be the first news-bringer.

"Mummy, Mummy," said Jacqueline, "imagine, there are three big lions very near by! The washgirl saw them this morning and she came to tell us. You're right, we don't have to go to the Kruger Park to see animals. We can see them from Auntie Sue's house. Oh, thank you, Auntie Sue, for living here, among the lions!" She added with glee, "Wait till I tell my friends, they'll be green with envy."

That clinched it. We settled on a compromise, involving less cycling and more car-transport, but they did stay on, and I believe that my sister caught some of the excitement herself.

The first victim was brought in to me that afternoon, a small fox terrier who had scented the lions while out with the farmers on the lion-hunt; it was hoped to destroy the intruders before they killed any more cattle. The dog followed spoor and actually pounced at the huge-maned giant, who at first ignored him, but then turned his head and threw him backwards, impaling him on the deadly canines before flinging him into the thorns. I did what I could for the little hero, but as he was so small, the tear-wound had penetrated deeply, and before I had gone very far with the repair-operation he expired, the bravest little dog I have ever handled. This whole episode sobered the children considerably, and their respect for predators at large increased; this was excellent, since in their eagerness to find lions they might otherwise have been tempted to break the rules that we had imposed. The lions were followed for many days and finally one of them was shot fatally; the other two disappeared into the heavy vegetation and the rocks, perhaps preferring a leaner sanctuary where prey was hard to come by in that rainy season, to the land of bovine plenty where they had been made so unwelcome. (During the dry season the game which the lions hunt become easy quarry since they have to come to collective watering places. In the rainy season, however, when pools of water abound, the predators' meat supply becomes more uncertain as their prey is widely scattered having no need of the regular water holes.)

Looking back on those days and months and years, I realise that my sister, though putting forward a city face on many occasions, actually helped me a great deal; we enjoyed many hilarious hours together. Sometimes, if I was hard pressed, she assisted me; once when I had to grapple with a human and an animal patient simultaneously she helped me nobly, though it was well after midnight.

Mr. Palmer was a tall, handsome farmer, a bachelor at the time; he had a wonderful bond of friendship with his white bull-terrier, which he called Zunda. This magnificent dog was one of the few which have been completely controlled by their masters; he was beautifully trained, his courage matched the reputation his breed enjoys, and he had a bright intelligence, which bull-terriers do not usually possess. Just before midnight in midwinter this farmer telephoned to inform me that Zunda had been ripped badly by a baboon, and that he would be more than grateful if I could help at this late hour. I told him to come at once, rose from my sleep-ridden state, washed and dressed and prepared for an operation as fast as I could.

"What now, in heaven's name?" mumbled my sister without stirring, "going out again?"

"Case coming in," I replied, though I felt that she was quite beyond hearing. "Bad baboon-injury."

"Nothing but wild animals in this place," she muttered dreamily. "Something must be wrong. I have always wanted to keep out of their way, and here I am right among them." With those words she once more sank into complete oblivion; I left, turned on the searchlight in the driveway and opened up the surgery.

Very soon – far too soon, I thought, considering the distance that Mr. Palmer must have covered between the time of his telephone call and the sound of his engine – I heard an approaching car; and within moments the precious white bull-terrier was lovingly placed upon the table. "Perhaps you should wait outside," I suggested, "I can call my orderly, he sleeps on the farm."

"Thank you, but no," replied the young man, "I am used to seeing wounds and I would like to stay and assist you, if I may." Within fifteen minutes the dog was shaved, cleaned, anaesthetised and covered in sterile cloths. We scrubbed up, gowned ourselves from the ever-ready steam-pressurised drum, and set out the instruments carefully on the sterile cloths. "All set?" I asked. "All set," he answered. The extent of the wound was terrible; as usual, the baboon must have bitten and pushed away his opponent in one single strong movement, judging by the exposure of peritoneal cavity and the length of the tear. The dog slept blissfully, breathing well, and deeply; and as I made my first incision I became aware of another kind of breathing superimposed upon the dog's. But I continued, intent on my work.

Crrrrash! My client had collapsed, and the hand holding the tissue forceps had disappeared. After the initial bump there wasn't much sound, and I was hard put to know what to do next. There was considerable haemorrhage, and I had to work fast to stem it and to repair the injured tissues, as well as watching the breathing and general behaviour of the dog. "You all right?", I asked foolishly, not taking my eyes or hands off my work. "Can you get up?" "Sorry, no," came the weak rejoinder, "but I have my head between my knees." Whenever I operated I kept a mobile bowl next to my elbow filled with sterile solution, into which I

SONGOLOLO IN MY BED

occasionally dipped my hands. I now gathered a handful of this and threw it across the table in the general direction of my fallen client, and was glad to hear a responding gasp. This really was a difficult situation. I supposed vaguely that since we live in a predominantly human world I should attend first to the farmer; he might be suffering from a heart attack. I swept this thought aside and gradually managed to convince myself (though my thoughts were disrupted by my intense activity and the late hour of the night) that my first duty as a veterinarian lay with the patient and that a dog-less owner was worse off than an owner-less dog.

At last the most difficult part of the operation was completed. I seized a sterile cloth, grabbed the extension telephone and turned the handle. I heard a heavy breathing sound and spoke. "Is that you, sis? Could you come up here and help me? – sorry to wake you!"

"No," said the voice, "the doctor is out, don't know where, I think she's attending a baboon. Better phone tomorrow."

"Hey, Alice," I almost yelled into the receiver, "it's me, Sue, your nutty sister, I need help badly, *please* pull yourself together."

"Okay, okay, you needn't speak so loudly, I can hear you. What's the trouble?"

"It's a man, a client, he seems to have passed out."

"Why didn't he go to the doctor in the first place! All right, I'll be there as quickly as I can."

With a sigh of relief, I returned to my dog, and some minutes later was relieved beyond words to hear light footsteps coming up the garden path.

The night ended well, after all, with Alice reviving a shamefaced farmer with coffee, and a successful outcome to the operation. We celebrated over the kitchen table until about three o'clock, when I suggested that we might all get some sleep and that I be kept informed early the next day of the dog's progress. "Not too early," pleaded my sister, "I'd love to be able to catch up with some sleep."

Fortunately Mr. Palmer had no need to call me until much later that day, and in fact I did not see my patient again until the following week. Then I had to remove the vast number of stitches I had put in and also to X-ray him for a suspected porcupine quill in the shoulder region, sequel to a fight he had obviously enjoyed the previous day, when he should have been convalescing. The quill did in fact show up, and this resulted in another hour on the operating table: I managed to find the broken-off shaft deep in the shoulder muscle. On this occasion my client did not volunteer to watch or assist, but withdrew discreetly to his car and left it all to us. "Please do thank your sister very much for her help," he said as he drove off for the second time, "one can easily see that she is a great lover of all animals, no fear of anything."

Although the children had persuaded the family to stay through the entire lion episode, which my sister had braved in the manner becoming to an ex-Norland war nurse, two things occurred which finally caused the departure of the city tribe. I had again been working late, and Alice had gone off to read in bed, wishing me good night and hoping that my cat-case would not keep me too long. I had just finished and was closing the surgery windows, when I heard loud screams and saw the children come running up to me from the house. "It's Mummy!" cried Ian, "she has a black snake in her bed; please come and help, before Mummy faints." I hastened towards the house in some alarm, snatching a big stick from the hall-way as I entered. As I opened the bedroom door an amazing sight met my eyes. Alice was precariously balanced on top of the bookshelf brandishing my How-to-Keep-Fit book, obviously very frightened though not yet hysterical. "Do something!" she said, "I think there is a black mamba in my bed. I just hope I haven't been bitten!" I did not wish to worsen matters by telling her that if she had been bitten by a mamba she would be dead in three minutes! I tried to keep a level head by convincing myself that with seven snake-catching cats and a gauzed-in house there was hardly any chance of a snake entering a bedroom, much less a bed. Very gingerly, holding my stick in one hand, I levered the covers farther and farther back while my heart hammered in my throat. Just as I was getting bolder and deciding that all this had been imagination, I saw a black Songololo (thousand legs) on the sheet. "It's quite harmless," I said with relief, "when I touch it, it will curl up." As I touched the creature with the stick it curled into a tight ball; I picked it up and put it on the lawn.

This was a terrible trial for Alice; although we laughed about it together for years afterwards, at the time it created quite a lot of nervous tension. "I'm just a bundle of nerves, after all, and I can't help thinking that maybe next time it *will* be a snake. Perhaps we had better go tomorrow."

Next morning, as the family was packing up, they discovered that most of the newly-laundered underwear was missing, and we stopped packing for some time to search for it. Finally we consulted Sam and, as usual, he had the answer. "Didn't want to tell you, madam," he said, smiling, "but Lucky, she ate your panties. I told Petrus you would soon find out, and it was his fault for not keeping her away. I hope madam will not go because of Lucky being hungry?"

"Well, no, Sam," Alice said kindly, "it is really time for us to go anyway. Perhaps next time we come, you will put a fence round the washing line. I'm surprised there weren't some bits of lace and elastic in the morning milk!"

We parted lovingly and with regret, as we always did; our existence was somewhat more earthy than theirs in the city, and I suspect that these weeks with us offered them that change and contrast without which life loses its piquancy.

CHAPTER 10

Caesarian in the Sun

Lucky had joined our family circle many years previously. It had all begun one midday, as hot a midday as one can get in the Lowveld midwinter, which is very hot indeed. A call had just been relayed to me from a farm eight miles away in a little village called Plaston; a tiny place, boasting one church, one post office, two garages, and a few proud inhabitants who deeply resent it when their little village is included within the White River municipality.

I was called there to an urgent calving case: the mother was unable to produce her calf, which was to prove oversize. By the time I reached her she was exhausted, unable to stand and obviously in pain. After a brief examination, I found that her uterus was completely inert, and concluded that this was a clear case for Caesarian section. Gone are the days when vets struggled for hours trying to deliver malpresentations (abnormal birth presentations), cutting them up internally and removing them piecemeal. This process required great skill and practice, and if done by other than an expert it often resulted in injury and a doubtful breeding future for the cow.

As we walked down the slope in the blazing sun, laden with equipment, I wistfully visualised the Caesarian section I had witnessed in a human operating-theatre not so long before. I recalled with longing the cool efficiency of the hospital, the well-trained nurses and sister, the surgeon's skill, the attentive anaesthetist and assistant surgeon. I mused on the difference between our labours, a difference so vast that it must be seen to be believed. I was about to operate on a recumbent cow, to be anaesthetist, nurse, and surgeon all at once; and, most important, I had to rally lay helpers and provide them with cheer and moral support, for without them such an operation was impossible. The reaction of the average person, even country-bred, to the sight of blood is always unpredictable; and for this reason I summoned every available hand on the farm, white, black or coloured, knowing that only a quarter of them or so would stay upright during the lengthy procedure.

We finally found the patient at the bottom of a rugged, shrub-covered hill, having walked at least three-quarters of a mile. It was a hot, dry and thirsty day, and I had, as usual forgotten to bring my hat. The only water we had with us was in the sealed bucket, and even this was now in solution with surgical soap – not the most appetising beverage, even when one is parched and hot. The only other fluid available was that in the cow's drinking drum, and this resembled a murky and stagnant pond. I threw myself into the job in hand, which is always a good cure for hopeless cravings: soon I had made the first incision. The prelude to this stage – which often brings the downfall of such willing helpers as are allergic to squirting arteries and the sound of a scalpel hissing on gaping flesh – takes about half an hour: local anaesthetic solution is injected into the spinal canal between the first and second coccygeal (tail) vertebrae, and while this takes effect the site of the operation is clipped and sterilised. Normally, when the animal is standing, she will lie down in about ten to fifteen minutes. There is no struggle and no need for ropes: the whole process is much quieter and infinitely safer than using a general anaesthetic.

As this cow seemed to be paralysed, we waited for a little longer to make certain that the full effect had been achieved. She was by now lying on her side, offering no resistance, looking at us with doleful eyes, much calmer since her stress and discomfort had been dispelled by the spinal anaesthetic. At this stage I did not know that she had not risen for several days; the owner had not seen fit to confide in me. This happens often, and of course, a full history sometimes makes a tremendous difference in the treatment of a case. It is a common failing of clients to mislead their vet; one reaches a stage where one hardly ever accepts anything that one is told. This creates a vicious circle; the scepticism produces suspicion, and much time and temper can be wasted in consequence. An owner will often feel guilty for calling in the vet at such a late stage, and invent all sorts of ridiculous stories to explain the present and often desperate state of his animal. After some years in practice, most vets develop a sixth diagnostic sense of their own, which enables them to be realistic in relating an animal's case-history, as told to them, with the visible facts.

There are many different methods of performing a Caesarian section; my preferred site is the area immediately in front of, and right-lateral to, the udder. My incision was about fifteen inches long, and it brought no muscular or general response since I had taken the extra precaution of injecting local anaesthetic solution into the deep muscle-layers and skin as well as epidurally (into the spinal cord). The muscle-layers were divided, clamped, held with tissue-forceps by my orderly and the other helpers, and not released until much later. As soon as I had opened the peritoneum, the uterus became visible underneath, bulging and distended, alive with its foetal burden. I had directed two of the more intelligent helpers to stand at the ready with sacks just behind my right shoulder, ready to receive the calf.

My orderly had meanwhile relinquished his forceps to another pair of hands and scrubbed up in the strong surgical soap without any prompting from me. As soon as the uterus was exposed, he immersed his arms carefully and skilfully into the peritoneal cavity, helping me to bring the uterus to the incision site and maintaining it there while I packed it off with sterile cloths and large gauze-covered swabs, prepared specially for this kind of work. For a fleeting moment I glanced round the gathering, trying to detect if there were any signs of imminent collapse which might hamper delivery. "It is all right, Doctor, *lungili*," said Sam, reading my thoughts as usual, "every one strong and awake." With one sweeping movement I cut the least vascular portion of the uterine wall for six inches and as I did so the uterine fluids poured out, drenching everything, but channelled away from the abdominal cavity by the tightly-packed material. The calf's left leg was there, tucked against the right; these were easy to grasp, and slowly I eased out the large, wet body and handed it to the waiting hands of the African behind me. He immediately took over, vigorously dried and rubbed and slapped the newborn, until at last it gave a long low bellow of protest. I gave a sigh of relief and prepared to sew up, a task which was arduous and slow and much less exciting than the initial part of the operation. "Take over now," the surgeon had said in the human operating theatre, and he had left the rest to his assistant. Even so, I

CAESARIAN IN THE SUN

would not have changed places with that streamlined human doctor; for through those back-breaking hours, through that dust-filled sun-baked atmosphere, there throbbed a rhythm of life and a challenge and closeness to the earth, which has long since been lost in the cool efficiency of green gowns and reflecting mirrors.

There were signs of life behind me, and I heard the Africans laugh. "It is a girl-calf," said Sam proudly, now released from his cramped position, preparing gut and needles for me as I stitched the different layers. "They say this girl-cow will be strong and naughty, for she is trying to walk already before her hair is dry." I glanced behind me and for a moment I saw the large brown body, which must have weighed at least seventy pounds, and the entrancing eyes, the muzzle, the velvet face. I have never outgrown my feeling of absolute awe and wonderment at the miracle of birth. One moment in the dark confines of pre-natal life, and the next in a bright new world, hard, strange and unfriendly.

It always took a full half-hour to sew up, and each time I wished anew that I had taken my mother's advice and learnt to use a thimble: the large circular cutting needles played havoc with my finger-tips. As I reached the final skin layer the calf must have got a whiff of the milk bar, for she suddenly staggered into the instrument tray scattering instruments, cloths, and swabs to right and left, determined to assuage her thirst, though the cow's supply was very poor after all her trials and tribulations. I was surprised to see the calf's strength, and allowed her to reach the teats while I carried on as best as I could to the finish, threading, snipping and stitching with renewed energy: the sight of the calf trying to drink had revived my own thirst, and I could think of nothing more wonderful than a long glass of cold milk.

After being in a half-kneeling position for one and a half hours, one's legs don't seem to respond to one's commands. As I tried to unbend and rise, I felt about a hundred years old – I had literally 'seized up', and it took me considerable time to rise from the sacks which had been kindly spread out for me on the ground, though by this time they were covered with a gory, sticky liquid. But that was all part of it. To be able to bring a healthy calf into the world – even one alive for every five delivered – gave immense satisfaction and joy, a feeling that in a so often destructive profession, there are times when one can be directly responsible for new life.

Most cows recover extremely well after this operation. They are up and grazing within two hours, and the milk supply does not drop very much at the beginning and after two weeks may even exceed all previous records. The stitches are removed in fourteen days, and the breeding cycle of the cow is, in most cases, undisturbed. This always amazed me, for the circumstances under which such a Caesarian section is carried out are very primitive. Dust and dirt cannot be prevented from entering the wound sites, and it is difficult, if not impossible, to maintain sterility under those circumstances. The bovine has a marvellous resistance to infection which surpasses that of any other species. Only very rarely does infection set in or any complication arise. But this was an exceptional case: the cow was unable ever to rise again and had to be destroyed.

I cannot imagine how we came into possession of this heifer calf, but we did, and the African's prediction came true: she was both lively and naughty from the day she entered our world. We raised her in company with the donkeys and dogs, and she thrived on substitute milk and human love. Her companionship with the donkeys was disrupted when the young foal bit off the end of her tail, just as a joke, thus marking her for the rest of time. She then very wisely concentrated on her canine friends, and seemed to think that she was actually of that species herself. This became more evident when the time came for her to seek the company of a Jersey bull. She was sent to a farmer friend and there put with a herd of cattle, which we thought would make her immensely happy. How little we knew about her! At the first sight of a pair of horns she tucked in her tail, put down her head and just ran, through fences, and orchards, down hills and valleys, horrified at the sight of her own kind. It took a great deal of time and patience to subdue her, and she was then brought back to be broken in more gradually; it took many months before she realised that she, too, looked like a cow.

When she returned to us she was in calf, and from then on she bore us much fine progeny, giving copious quantities of creamy milk for many years. She was never again sent away for mating, since she always broke out of the farm whenever she felt com-

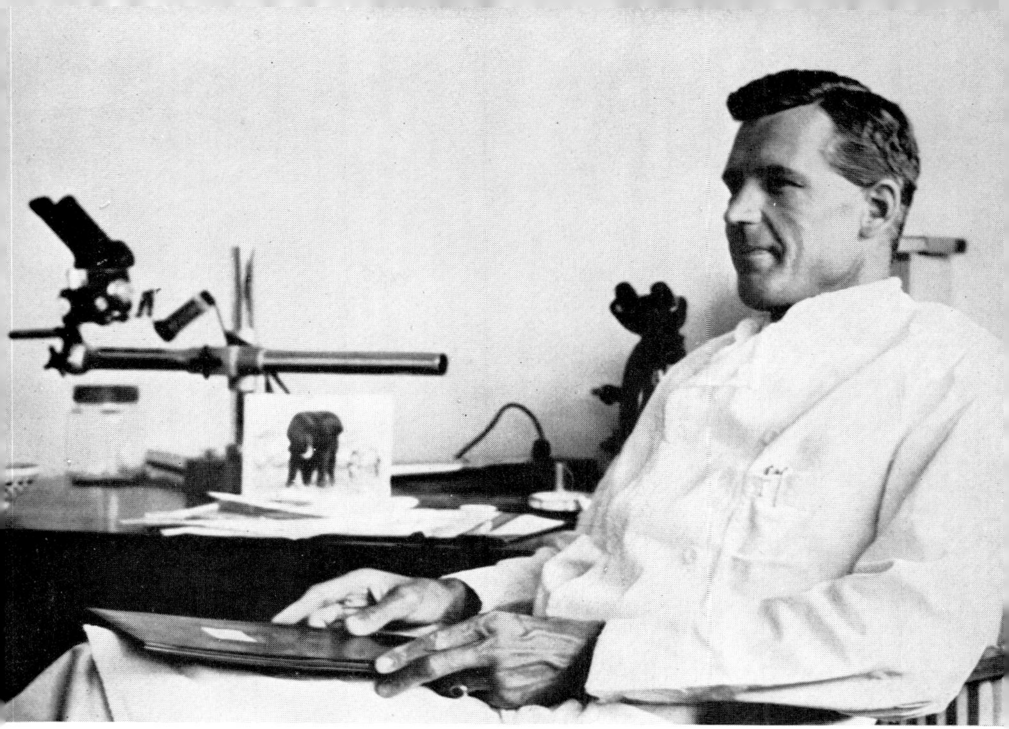

16. Toni Harthoorn in his "sanctum" at the University.

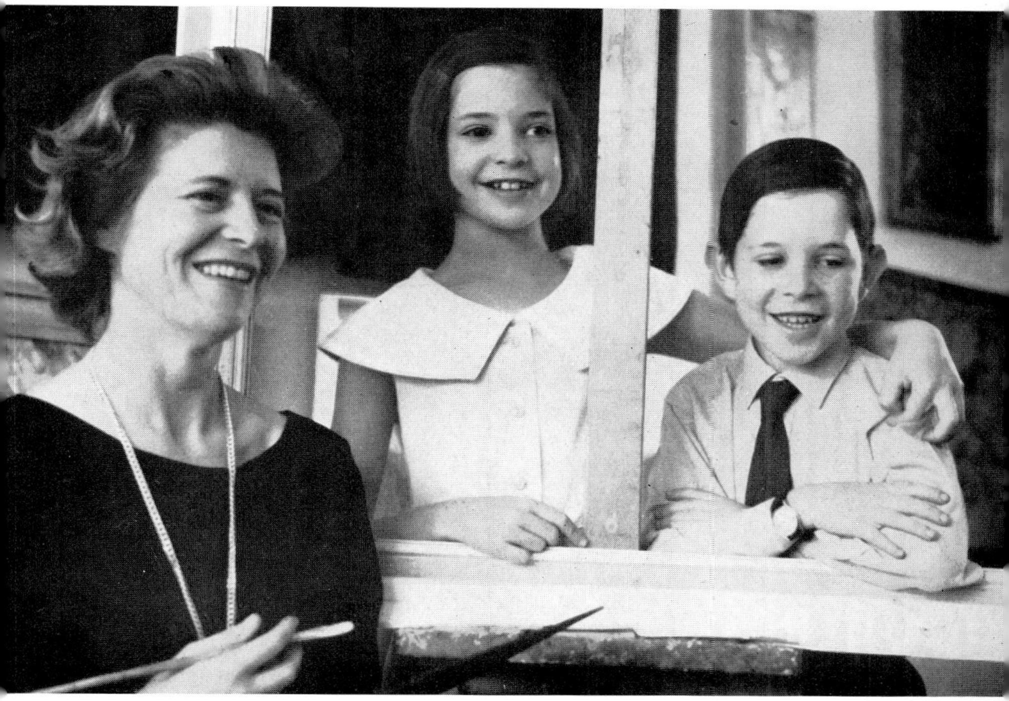

17. The author's sister, Alice, with her two children.

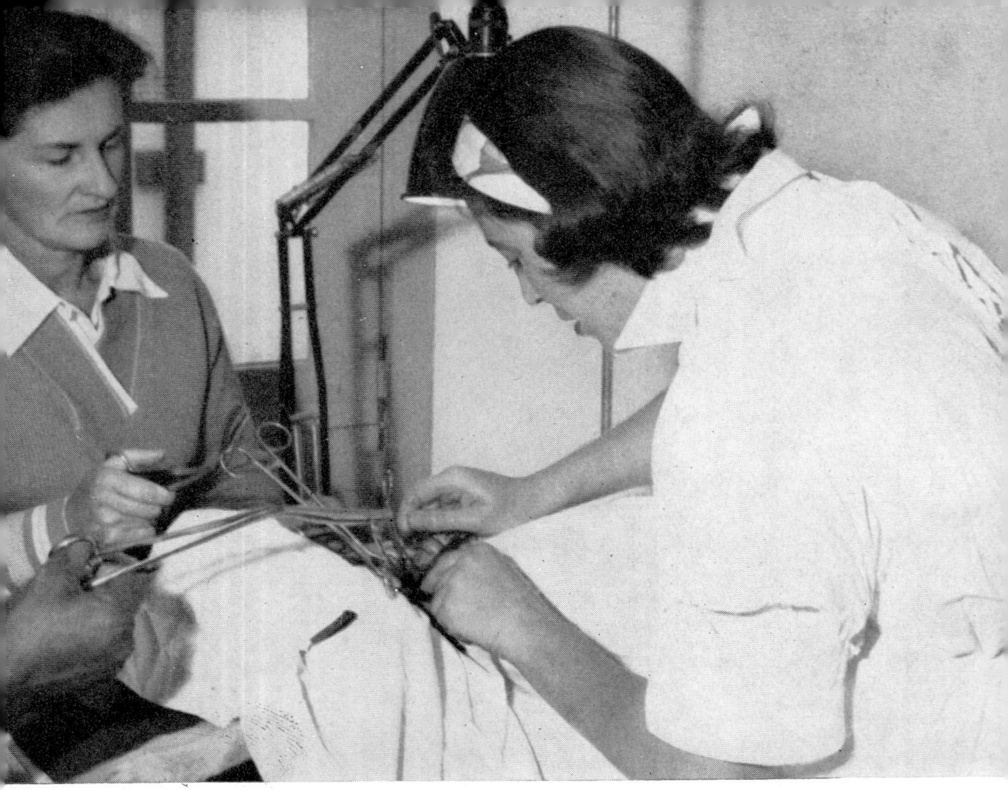

18. The author performing surgery with the help of her secretary and orderly.

19. The author and Sam with Lucky and Cheetah standing in front of the *kaaia*.

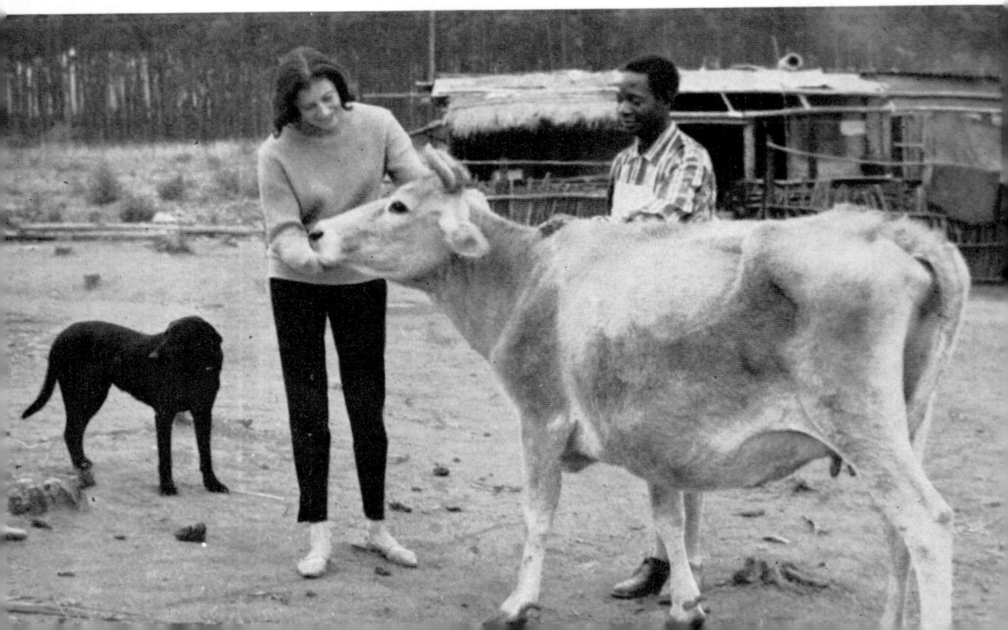

pelled to find a husband, returning only when it suited her, thus saving us a great deal of worry about the selection of a suitable bull and our transport and stud-fees.

On the day when we moved into the larger farm-house, she was left to her own resources in the new grounds and we neglected to feed her an extra ration at the accustomed time. Her retaliation was costly; she entered my bedroom through the open french windows, just after the furniture and carpet had been installed, and proceeded to consume my pink bedspread with relish. By the time she was discovered much of the damage had been done, and the pink rug was heavily fertilised with cow-dung.

Her taste for textiles persisted; after one year, during which she had eaten many jerseys and socks, much underwear and even parts of sheets, we decided to call it a day and fence off the garden from the farmland. This would be cheaper than paying endless compensation for guests' clothing. But occasionally some unwary person would still spread some washing delicacy upon the fence, rather than seek the revolving clothes-line, and in some uncanny manner Lucky would get the scent immediately and proceed to macerate it to shreds in a matter of minutes. I once found the new garden-boy having a tug-of-war with her over his blue overalls, which had already entered her mouth to the sleeve-shoulder seam on one side. Petrus finally won the battle and retrieved his garment – what was left of it – and wore the overalls proudly in this state from that time on, explaining to anyone who cared to inquire, that this was the result of a battle to the death with the *inkomo* of the doctor, a fearsome beast!

Lucky, our beloved and mischievous cow, became one of the characters of the district, joining the ranks of the two-legged oddities which abounded in our Lowveld. It would be difficult to name a location more variously coloured with odd people than ours, more marked by human eccentricity and diversity.

Often, when checking into hotels during our holidays, we have been surprised by the owner having some knowledge of our little village. On the Natal coast, one merry proprietor was absolutely delighted to welcome us; his face lit up as he recalled Lowveld memories, long before my time. "I know that place well," he said excitedly. "Mad as hatters they are there, or were in my day. What a collection! Hope they haven't changed." I assured him that we did indeed still cherish the proud spirit of his day, and proceeded to answer his many questions about inhabitants, past and present.

He had known two of the most famous characters in our area for many years, a pair of ladies affectionately called "the girls". They have lived for many years in a fertile valley above a lake known as Longmere, six miles from the village. They are as much part and parcel of our community as the huge umbrella-tree which stands in greeting on the roadside as one enters the low-lying valleys of the Lowveld at Alkmaar. They are a phenomenon, a rare thing – a partnership of two people as diametrically opposed as to make one wonder how they have managed to live together for so long. When they first came to the Lowveld many years ago, their visit was seasonal; each was an athletics coach, and they came to Africa mainly to escape the English winter, when sport was discontinued. Gradually the magic of those regions crept into their veins, and they decided to stay and build up a farm together. In a relatively short time this valley, known as Foresight, became one of the show places of the region; "the girls" specialised in horse-breeding and good cattle-management, but they also kept every other kind of animal, from rabbits to sheep, in true old English style.

Their livestock included a manager of male sex and immense courage, for he managed to stay for longer than one year, whereas his predecessors' days at Foresight had never exceeded one hundred and eighty. Since self-respecting farm managers don't like to be managed, a steady stream of them had come and gone over the years. This state of affairs was happily accepted by the two ladies, and their surprise must have been great when this ex-cotton-farmer and adventurer from Tanzania did not run to pattern, but survived the ordeal of working for two women who continually gave contradictory orders.

This young man, with his guitar, sang himself into the hearts of young and old, and soon became indispensable to his employers. He treated them as helpless females rather than as fearsome tyrants and very soon established a regular pattern whereby he gave notice whenever their manner became too aggressive; this caused them to become gentle and accommodating at once! Whenever we met, and I asked him how things were going, he would dryly reply either "Just given notice again!" or "Just about time to give notice!" Everyone admired him, for his ability to remain stemmed more from quiet humility and a bubbling humour than from cunning or tenacity.

The worthy pioneers for whom he worked not only had the most opposite characters possible, but appeared as physically different as Laurel and Hardy. One – long and thin, short hair, dressed in male garb – had a phenomenal capacity for work and a great devotion to the animal kingdom. The other – short and bulky, more dominant – was wholly dedicated to horses and whisky. They were the first women ever to drive from the Cape to Cairo; the first also to import valuable stud horses into this area where, not so long ago, equines could not survive the horse-sickness menace. Their mannish appearance was deceptive, and although they seemed well beyond the age at which girls are usually so called, I suspect that this joint title for them will be retained for posterity.

Soon after my advent into the Eastern Transvaal, a newspaperman published an extensive article dealing exclusively with the women who lived alone in the district, said to number forty-three at the last count. As the total white population does not exceed three thousand, this may have seemed rather a high estimate; but for my part I suspected that this figure was conservative. The type of woman attracted by the Lowveld in those early days was doubtlessly built of sterner stuff than her male counterpart.

Many of these lone ladies – some widows, some spinsters, and a sprinkling of divorcees – lived down a winding lane of great arboreal beauty known as 'Snobs' Alley'. Here also stood a fine outpost of the British Empire, dating back to the early days and aptly named the Planters' Club; this exclusive meeting-place of the English residents was at one time in great danger of falling into decay, but it was rescued and restored in the nick of time by a group of loyalists.

Many of my clients lived along this road, and at first, when my practice was in its infancy, I was very nervous of some of these ancients. Their manner was often offensive and brusque, their external personalities hardened by many years of command over their labourers.

On one of my first days of practice I was completely overwhelmed by one of these ladies; she descended upon me, dressed in black from umbrella to shoes, sweeping into my waiting-room and demanding that I immediately destroy no less than thirteen cats, who were beginning to become a nuisance to her. She eyed me with forbidding countenance, as if I had already earned her disfavour, and waited for my reply, tapping her cane on the floor. "You look far too young to manage anything," she said. "I had rather expected to find an older and more capable-looking woman." Until she made this remark I was in a state of only slight turmoil, for I was weighing my conscience against the dismissal of a new client. But when she attacked me in this ungracious manner, I decided to counter-attack, and my flagging spirits revived as I prepared for battle. I demanded why such a large number of cats should be destroyed; and I charged her with negligence, since it is easy to prevent the multiplication of felines. "I did not study all these years just to become a destroyer," I added finally, "and where I come from, such a case could be taken to higher authorities. Unless you have a sick cat or one beyond medical treatment, I cannot help you at all."

This last remark seemed to stop the black-clad lady in her tracks. She was obviously debating in her mind whether to walk out with a proud flourish of her umbrella, or stay and see the thing through. She decided on the latter, and broke – most unexpectedly – into a most charming smile, which shone under her stormy wide-brimmed hat like a sudden shaft of sunlight on a cloudy day. "Plenty of spirit you have, my child, for your young years. Come and have a drink with me tonight, and we will discuss this. Six o'clock!" She was gone before I could reply; and although I had, at that moment, no intention of keeping the appointment, by the time five o'clock came I knew that I would have to meet this challenge; and accordingly I made my way down 'Snobs' Alley'.

Great was my surprise when I found her seated in a blue-velveted chair among her cats and dogs, exuding kindness and tenderness, her home like something out of a fairy-tale, old-fashioned, full of trinkets and old books, gracious and harmonious, from the door-bell which rang heavily between the creeping ivy to the old broken-toothed heavily-wrinkled Zulu who brought the tray and bowed as he left the room. It was difficult to associate this gentle old lady with the fury who had demanded extermination of a whole tribe of felines only a few hours before. When she opened the subject again, just before it was time for me to leave, I found that she now had no intention of carrying through her threat; her earlier determination had only sprung from the fact that two of her cats had that morning brought two half-dead birds into the house, a sight which had inspired her to reckless action. In the end I did destroy two of the miscreants, for they were eczema-ridden beyond hope; and we found homes for six others, leaving only five. In the ensuing years I developed a great affection for the lady in black, and few weeks would pass without a visit to her, even if only for a few moments when passing. If I came before eight o'clock in the morning, I had to seek her out among the citrus trees, where she would be walking along the rows, inspecting the fruit and the labour force alike. By now she had reached the age of eighty years, and it seemed that nothing could stop her from going on until she made her century. If only the body could keep pace with the forward-looking spirit.

Almost directly across the road from her lived another very wonderful widow, Mrs. Farquhar, about twelve years older and fairy-like. The children, whom she loved and often invited, insisted that she was actually a fairy in disguise, and that she could have conjured up a wand and a star-spangled dress in the flick of an eye. She was usually to be found among her flowers, which ranged from sweet-scented roses to deep blue violets; whenever we called she was in her garden, facing the southern hills, her impish alert face and small fragile body framed among the long low branches of the heart-shaped bohemia leaves or pink blossom. She gave me much help with my teaching projects in African schools and she herself worked for many years among the needy, and not as a charitable pastime: she was a pillar of strength, the originator of many new ideas which came to be adopted and perpetuated in the Lowveld.

I was deeply moved when I heard, shortly before she died, that she wished to see me and reaffirm our mutual friendship for all time. She had passed in and out of a comatose state for some days, and we hoped, for her sake, that she might soon be able to pass on quietly without too much distress. On this last occasion when I visited her, she motioned to me to sit on her bed and grasped my hands, her dynamic spirit alive in her glowing lustrous eyes, her body barely tangible. "Tell me," she pleaded with short drawn breaths, "why is there so much unkindness and suffering everywhere? Is there really a reason for it all? Do you believe that we are re-incarnated?" She leaned back on her pillows and waited for my reply, her eyes searching mine as though to find the answer there. I felt that her need to know was great, and hoped that she would not be too exhausted; I had been warned to spend no more than a few moments with her, and these moments had already gone. "We have to suffer at the hands of others, for only in this way can we grow spiritually, until finally we need not return again to this world, our schoolhouse. The unkindness of others which has hurt you so much are only the growing-pains of pupils as they learn their lessons. We are all at different stages of development – some of us still at the beginning, thinking we know so much, and others near the final stage at which unkindness and suffering will not be able to hurt them further, for they know why it has to be. I am certain that we come back again and again; there is no other way in which we can pay the debts we have incurred and wipe our slate clean."

There was a soft knock on the door from Mona, the old lady's nurse and companion, whose humour and delightful personality had made her last months a gentle transition between life and death when they could have well been otherwise. She warned me that it was now time to leave, and so I took the last farewell of my elf-like friend with my eyes alone, for she had fallen asleep as I finished speaking. Twenty-four hours later she had gone, and we were happy to hear it: she had become impatient with her earthly home, and desired nothing but permission to leave it.

As I prepared to go, a telephone message reached me from the brickfields, where another snake-bite case apparently needed my urgent attention. My mind was still in that quiet little room as I sped along the Plaston road; I had to force myself back to veterinary reality, checking from memory the contents of my medical case and trying hard to remember how many doses of snake antiserum I had put into it that morning. I passed the railway crossing, thankful that it was empty of trains, and turned into the last lap before the brickfield track deviated from the main sand road. If this was going to be like the last time and the time before, all the serum in the world would do no good.

Friday was cattle-dipping day in the Lowveld, and on this day the herd was driven to the kraal (cattle enclosure) only two miles from the homestead. It was open hill country, wooded with wattles and gumtrees and sparsely planted with crops, giving enough grazing for about fifty cattle. This was the valley of the brickmaker, where the ancient method of using mules to turn the clay mixer was still used. In this remote back-country, inhabited only by a few kindly farmers, I always got the strange sensation that time stood still and that the outside world beyond the rock had left this place behind while it raced ahead down the years.

Only the deadly mamba knew the meaning of speed in this farmland and she had struck again with fatal effect, this time at an ox as he was being herded into the dipping enclosure. For the third time in three weeks I had arrived too late: the black beast lay, still warm but quite dead, at the entrance to the crush.

"Oh, Doctor, what shall we do now? We have tried to burn it, smoke it out and shoot it out, but this snake has an uncanny way to elude us. It appears, quick as lightning, strikes its victim and disappears again."

I examined the ox and found the usual evidence, on the leg this time. "Better admit defeat and move the dip tank; it will cost you less in the long run. Perhaps the snake has young and is protecting them."

"It is a monster spirit, *docotele*," said the head herdsman darkly, "we cannot come here again, for next time she may kill one of us."

And so the new kraal was built while the farmer had to bear the losses of three oxen and one cow and much extra expense besides. This was an unusual case, fortunately; in most instances the snake is not an aggressor, but a defender.

During the wet summer months snake-bite cases were an almost daily occurrence and I made it a routine to check over my snake-bite equipment before retiring at night. I did not carry less than six ampoules at one time but had to rotate these carefully between my case and the cooler, as great heat would eventually cause deterioration of the serum. I had been told, when arriving in the Lowveld, that snakes were hardly ever seen and rarely bit anyone. Perhaps this was true of some areas, but within our own area snake damage occurred frequently. Many native herd-boys, walking barefoot through the fields, fell victim, often to the puff-adder. When I visited the Swedish Mission Hospital for Africans, where my X-rays were done, I was always amazed and horrified to find how many snake-bite cases were under treatment there at one time.

In my own sphere of work the large breeds of dog were the ones most often bitten, since they are slow and aggressively playful, and would follow a fleeing snake into the undergrowth until it turned and attacked them in pure self-defence. The puff-adder, which is slow to move and the snake most commonly encountered, usually bit the face or muzzle, and by the time the dog was brought to me the appearance of the head would make diagnosis easy. The brachiocephalic types (such as the bulldog and boxer) would by now resemble prehistoric monsters rather than dogs; the swelling, which covered most of the face and neck, was board-like and hard in the initial stages.

At first I had little success in cases which arrived in an advanced stage, but gradually I discovered that dogs would tolerate far more snake anti-serum than humans. Up to this time I had based the treatment on that given to human patients; my new therapy had more success. I increased the number of ampoules, given intravenously at four-hourly intervals, and provided at the same time dextrose and other anti-shock treatment: my survival rate increased by fifty per cent in the first snake season. Much depended on the condition of the animal which was bitten, and also its breed; small dogs needed larger doses of serum, relative to their size, and if they belonged to the 'toy' type of overbred dog their chances were far less than if they were good hardy mongrels. My neighbour's own dog, a cross-bred ridgeback, died within ten minutes of being bitten by a ringhals, another species of adder; he breathed his last as he was placed on my surgery table. This dog had been playing with the snake, together with his litter mate, who was no less fierce than he; and as the snake had attacked one dog, the other had bitten her clean in half. In that split second, the snake had curled back and struck at the second dog's lip, revenging itself as death overtook it.

On the whole, smaller breeds do not get bitten so frequently; they are more agile, and they seem to know when to stop the game and when the moment is favourable to a kill. Cats are the most successful snake-killers of all, with the exception of the mongoose, and for this reason I kept no less than seven cats round the farm, hoping that they would prevent reptiles from entering the house and lurking in the garden. Our black tom cat excelled himself when he was barely six months old by keeping a deadly night-adder at bay for twenty minutes, while the snake was furiously attempting to find a vulnerable spot in the defence. I wanted to interfere; but Sam, standing by, assured me that our cat would be the victor, and that by stopping the fight I might cause the snake to gain the upper hand, even for a split second. I noticed that after some time the snake became slower in its movements, and that the evading action of the kitten had changed its rhythm. Suddenly, so fast that I only saw fur flash across my line of vision, the cat counter-attacked; and within seconds it was all over. He had bitten the snake neatly behind the head and was only waiting for the coils to cease their movement. "You see, madam doctor, I told you it is best to leave alone, *okati* (the cat) always knows best!" And Sam went back to the kitchen, nodding his head with satisfaction.

CHAPTER 11

The Potter's Hand

My family was worried when they heard of the daily perils of my life. I never mentioned any of the more dangerous tasks that I had to perform, but news of my activities nevertheless filtered through to the city – though how this happened, when the distance was so great, I shall never understand. Mother telephoned us shortly after the snake incident, sounding worried and tense. "You told us that one never sees snakes in the Lowveld; and now you have them in your back garden, a whole nest of them. I do think you should move from the farm into the township as soon as possible; I will come and help you." I tried to reassure her but she was not to be bluffed. "Your father will be down tomorrow to speak to you about it; it's not only you, it's the children we are worried about!" Poor Mother! – from the very beginning she had to put up with my eccentricities, as my sister called them, and being now within telephone distance made matters much worse: well-meaning friends were always telling her about my latest adventure. "I hear she had to go and shoot a really vicious dog last week," one dear lady crooned at my horrified mother, "I just don't know what we would do without her." "Surely you don't really have to go out and *shoot* animals?" she said to me later, "that's a man's job!" I quite agreed with her; but unfortunately, since I had put up my veterinary plate, there wasn't anything which I could refuse to do. My own feelings didn't really enter into it. I had taken some lessons from a friend on how to handle a pistol, how to shoot and how to clean it, for this was my first experience of firearms. I never became a very good shot, but proficient enough to be able to effect destruction when I had to, though I liked this part of my work less than any other.

I had been called out late one evening to destroy a horse on one of the hill farms. This was the first time I had ever been requested to shoot an equine, and I dreaded the task: somehow, the destruction of such a noble creature seems far more terrible than destruction of any other animal. He was a grey gelding of great age, yet his thin body and scraggy legs held a dignity and a proud carriage that spoke of happier times. His only crime was his age and the fact that his worn-down teeth had become almost ineffective. This was the onset of the dry winter months, always the most trying season for grazers, and his owners had decided that precious pasture was wasted on him. We led him away from the house and I shot him next to his already-dug grave. It was all over in the crack of a pistol-shot, yet for me it was a most nauseating experience; and I drove home in the failing light, wondering if the job I had taken on was more than I could chew.

As I lay in bed that night I felt many misgivings about my life, and wondered how long I would be able to go on working for an uncaring, hard-baked public, whose greatest thought was for economics and not for the welfare of their animals. I remembered my parents' anxiety when I cast aside all their offers to send me to medical school, dramatic college, the school of music, anything but the veterinary college! I saw, again, my father's rosy face turn ashen grey as he watched me performing the unladylike rectal pregnancy diagnosis, my arm immersed into the rear end of the cow up to the shoulder. "Is *this* what you have learnt to do all those years at college? Just *this*?" Poor Dad, he really had no stomach for cow-dung! Fifteen years before, he had announced the fact that I wished to devote myself to this profession to my headmistress, and she had been surprisingly sympathetic. "I don't know what to do," Dad had lamented, "but my daughter insists that she wants to be a wet!" His Austrian accent had rather nonplussed Miss Edwards but she had, in good time, discovered what it was he had referred to. "For what you are doing, my pronounciation is better anyway," Dad often said when coming on calls with me. "I have never known a profession where one is wet so often!"

It was long after my father had thus startled the head of my school and when I had been practising for some years, that a friend and colleague came down to the Lowveld to help with some difficult cases. I was particularly glad to see him, as I was tired and still suffering from the after-effects of a course of anti-rabies treatment that I had just completed. "You should think about giving up soon," he had advised soberly, "this type of practice really takes it out of you. Give up before you have to." But I had already had an inkling that soon – within a year anyway – I would be giving up this work I loved, and that total collapse wasn't going to be the reason. At that time, my instinct only told me the outcome; the way in which I was to be taken away from this work had not been revealed. It had never occurred to me that I might re-marry and join forces with one of the most outstanding veterinary scientists of our time, and that his work would become my interest and my new sphere of activity.

"How could you have exposed yourself to active rabies?" my friend now asked with deep concern. "You are supposed to behave like a seasoned practitioner, you have even been proposed as a member of the Veterinary Council, and now I find you acting like an unfledged, foolhardy student!" There was truth in what he said, for I took far too few precautions; but then no practising vet can coddle himself with masks and gloves – one is far too busy to think of one's self. Yet complacency often leads to trouble, as I was to find to my cost, and a little jolt often brings one to one's senses.

The head of the veterinary institution reacted just as violently when I phoned him in a distraught state to seek his advice. I told him what had happened, and he was so outraged at my stupidity that he blew his top, so that I had to hold the telephone receiver some distance from my ears to prevent temporary deafness. "You mean to tell me that you put your ungloved hand down the dog's throat, when he had all the symptoms of an early rabies case? You must be out of your mind. I would fail any final-year student for much less than that!" The trouble was that many dogs seem to have the same symptoms in the early stages of distemper-like diseases, including encephalitis. I had given this dog a routine examination, which included a good look at his mouth and throat; and had I not had an open scratch on one of my fingers, all this fuss might have been avoided.

I prescribed the necessary medicines, or so I thought, and gave directions about treatment and care, and asked the owner to keep me informed of his progress or otherwise. "Please keep in touch with me, even if the dog improves and recovers quickly. I *must* know what happens to my patients after they leave me." Unfortunately only very few clients ever carried out this request, and many case records were thus made incomplete and useless. In this case, I heard nothing more for four days; and even at my busiest I had the uncomfortable sensation that there was something that I had to do which I could not quite recall to memory. At last I sat down and leafed through my diary, and eventually reached the relevant page; it made me sit up with a start, for I knew at once that something must have gone wrong with that patient. "Dead or better," my secretary used to say as consolation when we did not hear from our clients, and so it usually turned out to be.

This particular dog had been dead for two days by the time I had tracked down the owner. "Sorry I did not let you know, Doc, but I have been so busy planting. The dog was getting worse and began to behave very strangely, so I thought it would be safer all round if I shot him." My heart sank as I asked him to describe exactly what happened. "On the day after you saw him, he began to growl at us and skulked under chairs and in dark corners, which wasn't a bit like him. He wouldn't eat or drink, and when I fondled him he tried to bite me. Just seemed kinder to put him out, so I shot him after dark, when all the family were inside, and buried him deep, since it's so hot. Sorry I didn't let you know, Doc." "Had your dog been injected against rabies?" I asked, for this was my last hope. "Oh, yes," came the cheerful reply, "two days before he got so ill." That was it; my fear was justified. The vaccination could not have taken effect within such a short period of time. Worse still, it was doubtful whether a recently-injected dog which had died of rabies could ever have this deadly virus-infection confirmed pathologically, or in any other way – especially if it had to be removed from a grave in the midsummer Lowveld.

"I am afraid I will have to phone the veterinary headquarters at Onderstepoort to receive instructions; please dig up the body as soon as you can and bring him in. I am afraid otherwise we might be in trouble." I did not add that I knew quite well that we were already in trouble; I thought there was no point in alarming the poor man unduly before I had spoken to the powers that be.

"But, Doc," I heard him say, "it's so hot, it'll be a terrible messy job."

"Sorry about that," I commiserated, "but this may be rabies which falls under government jurisdiction anyway."

I managed to place an urgent call, and reached the Director of Veterinary Services within a few minutes. His reaction to my sad tale was anything but encouraging, and by the time I had the dog's brain safely stowed in my station-wagon and was making my way up to Pretoria, I felt more like a vet student who had just failed his final examinations than a qualified practitioner. I had contacted the local district surgeon and given him the complete history, so that the owners of the dog could also receive treatment, if he thought it necessary. They had handled the dog until the very end, and it was possible that some saliva had touched them; very few farmers can honestly say that the skin on their hands is completely unbroken, even by a minute cut or a broken blister.

I reached the research institute within six hours of my conversation with the director. It was too late to receive the protective serum which is often given while a diagnosis is tested and confirmed biologically and pathologically; the safety limit for this is seventy-two hours. "The injections you will have to undergo are very risky; there has been a case of paralysis quite recently, a medical doctor who had been bitten by a rabid pet mongoose. I admit there is a chance that you have been contaminated; but it is remote, and you must think carefully before you allow the health department to start on you." I set off to the city to consult the health department, and found them very helpful and cheering; but their doctor, charming as he was, made no bones about the fact that if I did *not* undergo the injections, I might end up as a foaming maniac! Memories of San Michele came to me, and it wasn't difficult to make up my mind which risk to take.

Fortunately I was able to spend this time at my sister's home in the hills of Waterkloof; and although the cause of my journey only confirmed what she already felt about my lunatic way of life, she was a tower of strength and gave me the moral support I needed. "Within six months you will know whether the injections are effective, or maybe before. If you feel well in another half-year, then you know you are safe." I had been warned that I should report the slightest untoward symptom – such as a tingling of a hand or foot, or any nausea or headache – and that I must see the doctor in charge of this section daily and receive my injection from him. The Lowveld family, or part of it, also had to undergo this treatment, and I kept track of them during my stay in the Highveld.

After I had received my eighth injection, by which time my stomach was beginning to look like an inflated pincushion, I was driving back into the hills when I felt a strange sensation in my left arm, travelling down to my hand on the steering-wheel. After some minutes I could feel no strength in my fingers, and I decided to continue the drive with my right hand alone. I informed the doctor-in-charge on my return, and he advised me to miss my next injection, and to call him should there be any further deterioration. By the next day the numbness had almost passed, and I wondered if I had imagined it; but the injections were stopped altogether, to my intense relief, and I was told to stay away from work for two weeks. I was four injections short, nothing to worry about, for an immunity must have been built up to some extent already.

I stayed for two more days, and then decided to return home and carry on with work – which would be, after all, the best distraction and antidote to worry. At this point, my colleague arrived to help me out; I found out later that he had already heard about the rabid dog, and had made up his mind to tempt me into a research post, before it was too late owing to some further foolishness of mine. "The law of averages holds good in every walk of life. You have been lucky; get out of practice, before your luck changes!"

Shortly after he left, my luck did begin to change; I was forced to admit that my guardian angels were busy elsewhere.

The first trouble was between myself and a huge Afrikander bull; it ended in the juiciest black eye imaginable, the envy of any boxer. I was called in to find out why the bull was impotent; he must have sensed somehow what was about to happen, for his behaviour was as recalcitrant as his manner was unwelcoming. In order to examine him minutely, we had first to inject an intravenous tranquilliser which would relax him from top to toe and make the examination easy to carry out thoroughly. There was no crushpen on this farm, so he had to be thrown, and for this procedure every pair of available hands was collected – from the orchards, from the gardens, from the planters – even the little piccanins came to see the fun and pretend to help. It was simple to put the ropes on him and bring him gently down, and I thought that the battle was won before it had actually started. I put the rope-ring round his neck to bring up the vein, and into it directed my newly-sharpened needle, when he suddenly twisted his great head and rapier horns and in one movement threw off the restrainers who were hanging on to him by the score. Perhaps they just dropped everything and ran; it was hard to know, for from my own vulnerable position alongside the curved back-neck, I could see very little, except a multitude of stars and bright lights as I was pitched into the long grass many yards away.

As I opened my aching eyes I noticed that the shamefaced crew were trying to recapture the half-breed bull, while exclamations of concern and pity for me flowed in and out of my temporarily distorted world. In the end I sedated the bull with an intramuscular injection, which took longer to be effective but was safer by far in the long run. I was sorry to find that he had to be condemned to the butchery; he was a magnificent specimen, but his condition was beyond repair, since the owner had waited too long before getting an opinion. My own peculiar facial appearance persisted for several weeks and I had to invent a good story so that my mother, who came to visit me during that period, would not be unduly alarmed. I simply told her that I walked into a stable beam, blinded by the transition from sunlight to darkness; whereupon she smiled at me enigmatically, as though she was making a sincere attempt to believe the story, and reprimanded me for not being more careful. "Always dreaming," she mused, "I should think that a cowshed could be a very dangerous place to dream in!"

Soon after my physiognomy returned to normal, I was asked to ring an obstreperous Guernsey bull, which should have been rung years ago before he became dangerous. He had already done some damage to a Zulu herd-boy, who had dived underneath the nearest cow for protection, this resulting in injury to the cow as well, for the ill-tempered bull had not been able to check his charge. He had chased and just missed numerous others, making himself thoroughly unpopular and becoming very much feared in the neighbourhood. The owner of the farm was overseas, but the young manager in charge had thoughtfully organised the building of a crush pen in order to protect me during the operation.

On this occasion I had a young male student with me; it was very early in the morning, and we drove up the last slippery farm road which led to the kraal and saw the bull standing among his harem. As we approached, I saw a young herd-boy climbing in, no doubt to hasten the herding process as he had been instructed. The events of the next moments passed so swiftly that I find it hard to recall every detail; something of what occurred left my memory completely, and I have had to reconstruct the episode partly from the accounts of others. As I opened our car door, I heard a terrible scream; racing to the fence, I saw that the little herd-boy had been attacked by the bull and was now pinned against the fence while the infuriated beast came at him again and again. My student was at the point of hysteria, and it took me a moment to sober him; then I saw Mike, the farm-manager, rushing up the hill alarmed by our shouts and together we leapt over that fence and down into the kraal, though how this was possible and why the bull turned away I cannot understand; we somehow dragged and half-carried the partly disembowelled body into safety and Mike and the shocked student heaved him into the back of my station-wagon, a moment after I had thrown out my boxes of equipment to make room for him. I drove as I have never driven before, though the boy, in full consciousness, pleaded with me in agonised tones to drive more slowly. This request I could not grant him, for I knew that every second was precious and that the mission hospital was over eight miles away. Had he been a European I am certain he would have lost consciousness at once, which would have been merciful. The Bantu are tough and more resistant to shock than we are, and it was not until he was on the operating-table that he sank into painless oblivion with the aid of an anaesthetic.

The staff of the hospital, almost entirely Swedish, were fast and efficient, taking everything in their stride, accustomed to all the horrors which can befall a man, white or black. Mike and I watched for a while, too stunned to move away, fascinated by the air of peace and harmony which reigned in that little operating-theatre, a striking contrast with the turmoil that we had just experienced. "Come outside, please!" Mike's voice was urgent; when we reached the passage he explained to me that we had neglected one very important fact – we had warned no one of the bull's frenzied state, and perhaps by now, he would have claimed a new victim. At once we rushed back to the station-wagon and once again I drove full out, wincing at the thought of what we might find on our return. We stopped at the manager's cottage to pick up a rifle, and I agreed to take full responsibility for the destruction of the bull in the owner's absence. Great was our relief when we found that no one else had entered the enclosure; in fact there was no sign of human life at all. The cows stood as before, waiting to be milked, and the bull among them, still hot and frothing at the mouth.

One perfect shot and all was still. We left the fatal place and strengthened ourselves with tea in the farm-house cottage until our hands became steady and our knees stopped shaking. I had to continue the morning's work, and so did Mike: we parted as if in a dream, wishing that the morning had never been. The student had recovered himself at the hospital and had driven off to the nearest large centre to find more blood for transfusion. I often wondered whether a similar experience at his age would have affected my own determination to become a country vet! The boy did eventually recover, but only after many months. He never again took on heavy work, but thrived on gentle gardening tasks, and enjoyed the respect and awe allotted to him by his companions: they believed that one must be great indeed to be saved from the jaws of death as he had been.

I found it very difficult to erase this episode from my mind. Again and again that morning scene would come before my eyes with agonising vividness, and with it the smell of blood and the sounds of distress. In the end I decided to find some antidote, some soothing influence; and I realised with sudden clarity that there was one place, and one place only, where I could find the peace and perspective which would counteract the poison in my system. How could I have forgotten that sanctuary among the aloe-flaming rocks in the echoing valley, where lay the pottery of Esias Bosch, facing the hills which stood one behind the other until the eye found their highest point, Piggs Peak, the sentinel of Swaziland? Sias, as he was called, is one of the few master earthenware potters in the world; his whole heart and soul were expressed in his creations, which seemed to convey to the beholder the strength and the rhythm of the earth from which he derived his clay, while his exquisite decorations and glazes portrayed and captured the ethereal beauty and magic which man can only seek above. Sias is an idealist, a man who strives to preserve peace within his own sphere at any cost, whose greatest love is for the things of nature, the simple things of the universe. Here a materialistic, restless man would stop in his tracks for the potter exudes a stillness and harmony which no one can fail to sense. To come into his world from the outside offers one such a striking contrast that one can hardly tell where one truly belongs: it is like moving from a bubbling cauldron into a peaceful lake.

We were friends, his family and mine, and we were also neighbours; yet each time I visited this oasis I felt privileged, not only because I could go there whenever I wished, but also because I was always welcome. Nothing was so soothing to me as to sit and watch and hear his wheel as it turned, its even gentle hum giving forth some wondrous shape, sometimes so high that Sias would stand on a box to create the upper part. The throwing-shed was usually full of his art, some pots waiting to be glazed and fired, others drying, fresh from the wheel. Many finished bowls and cups and plates stood on the long table, their graceful contours full of personality, alive, reflecting a different mood at every hour of the day as the light changed its angle.

Sometimes he would pause for a moment to explain his latest glaze or decoration or to conjure up a new idea for the next firing of his kiln, which was heated with wood. We might share a cup of coffee from his home-made and generously-shaped cups; or perhaps we would go outside, and sit on the rocks, and discuss our aims in life, and then into our conversation would creep the ever present murmur of the Lowveld. Sometimes he would proudly show me his collection of rare aloes; and I might be fortunate to see his giant lobelia flower, leaning against the wooden wall for support, glorious for one day only, a strange contrast against the thorny succulent mother plant from which it arose.

"Take this bowl, it is reject!" he would say, with a gentle warming smile which meant: "we both know it is *not* a reject, but let us pretend it is, and then you won't mind accepting it." And he would press into my hand an iridescent glowing blue and white bowl which contained the miracle of a bird in full flight within its concavity, free as the air, proud to have been born out of the magical clay. Then it would be time to go again, and we would part; but it was always a happy parting. I would climb out of the valley, and Sias would return and lose himself in his labour of love, until the dimming light brought him out of the valley, too. I had come to seek solace and oblivion from the stark realities and cruelties of life, and I had found it here. I felt revitalised and much richer for having spent those moments in the potter's presence.

CHAPTER 12

Bottles on my Shelf

Having passed through a period of turmoil I entered upon a more tranquil phase, partly because I now became aware of the interest that the young took in my work. I had never before understood the depth of their sympathetic seeking after knowledge and their consequent ease of communication with the animal world. It seems that sophistication, distraction and the treadmill of daily life draw adult man away from his animal inheritance of simplicity, his chance of true companionship with animals. And so I loved to watch children and learn from them, for their absorption and devotion is a tonic. If I became their teacher, it was only because I was richer in words and experience, not in natural wisdom; and at the end I felt I had learnt at least as much from them as they had from me.

It all began with the collection of bottles which I kept on top of the instrument cabinet. One day, when I was doing a post-mortem on a cow which had died only a few hours previously, I discovered a four-month foetus in the womb, and took it back with me to show to the children. The perfection of the little body impressed me more than ever before, and I decided to try and 'pickle' it for posterity. The children were delighted by the infantile bovine shape in the bottle and had gazed at it for many hours, exclaiming with wonder as they recognised the little hoofs, the ears, the eyes, the minute tail. "It is absolutely fabulous," said Gail, "I am going to tell all my friends all about it." Several days later a car drove up, and one adult followed by a crowd of small boys and girls burst forth towards the waiting-room: they had come to see the baby calf which they had been told about. Their interest was so great that I decided to preserve every foetus I could, as well as the other tissues and items, such as cystic calculi (bladder stones), which I removed in the course of surgery. While adults often felt repelled by my array of bottles, the children felt quite otherwise and revelled in the background history which was attached to each bottle on a label. I carefully kept the entire uterus of a Siamese cat which had to be excised, exposing one foetus of the six completely, another partially, and leaving the rest within their protective membranes, thus demonstrating the relative size of each individual enclosing sac and the difference between this and its cushioned contents. The children, some very young, were quite fascinated by this exhibit and especially by the minuteness of each kitten, which was nevertheless a perfect model of a feline. The collection grew steadily, as did the number of my visitors: and soon I took them on in groups for afternoons at a time, especially during their holidays.

It was my neighbour, Power S. Dzungwe, who first suggested that I should teach in schools. He was the headmaster of the Bantu school, and I had spent many hours there with him, examining the arts and crafts, talking to the pupils, advising them on problems concerning their animals. They were shy at first, but since their teacher had no shyness they soon lost theirs, and they would crowd round me, listening to some tale I invented on the spur of the moment to demonstrate my point. "Doctor should come and give lessons," Power said one day, "give them in the classrooms. We will much enjoy this." We discussed the idea at some length with his wife, Muriel, and in the end he promised to get me a list of the Bantu schools in the area, fourteen in all, stretching for miles into the hilly native Reserve.

Much had then to be done, for our plan needed organising; the sanction of the school authorities, the district commissioner's permission for me to enter the Reserve areas, contact with the heads of the individual schools, information on how to reach them – all these things had to be arranged. Even more important, I had to find a way into the hearts of these children; their way of life, the native scale of values, the strength among them of ancient traditions would force me to put my subject before them in a very distinctive way. I needed help, and this would have to be found amongst those who were more familiar than I was with native habits and their language, and who would be prepared to sacrifice time to this adventure in education.

I had often been asked to speak on veterinary subjects in European schools but I had never given of my best in the respect of what the children really wanted. I lectured above their heads, explained their obligations to their pets, told a few amusing stories and went my way. With the advent of the 'bottles on my shelf' era, something stirred within me; I realised quite suddenly that I had a tremendous opportunity to awaken the slumbering interest which nearly all children have in animals, wild and domestic. I would now have to learn how to do this in the best possible way; and the only way to learn was to do.

While I was making contacts and gathering material for my proposed work in African schools, I began to lecture in the others. At first my attention was directed at the children's reactions to whatever material I presented; and very soon I found that whenever I brought one of our own pets along – a dog, cat, dove, guinea-pig, or bush baby – their shyness would melt away. I introduced a question-time, making this almost as long as my own talk, and I soon found that by the time the bell rang I had not covered half my intended ground. Often the teachers were present and joined in the questions, and it became obvious to me that much apparent thoughtlessness and cruelty stems from nothing but ignorance. My black labrador, Cheetah, who later became the hero of my nation-wide broadcasts for schools, was very much attached to a certain pigeon in our menagerie; and I often took them both along, to show the children that there is no such thing as inborn enmity except where animals and birds have to fend for themselves in the wild, and then it is a case of kill or starve. The children were enthralled by this conception, and out of it came many hours of discussions shaped by their longing to know more and more about wild life.

Time had always been a problem in my life; now with my practice continuing as before, each day was far too short for what I wanted to do. The teaching programme grew into something much bigger than I had at first envisaged. I found people who were willing to help and who knew some aspect of what we wanted to teach – care of the small and large domestic animals, for example, the protection of game, the care of the old animal or of birds and fish, together with first-aid demonstrations. We planned all this in such a way that each class of children should have two sessions a month dealing with alternate subjects: this gave them time to prepare questions in between. We co-ordinated our talks for the sake of continuity, and arranged to bring in live animals whenever possible, ranging from calves to owls and snakes. We had to fit in with the syllabus and general plan of the schools and submit our subject-matter for one year ahead. As we were in a bilingual country, we had to provide bilingual speakers; I was delighted to find that there was no shortage of naturalists and devoted farmers in both sections of the community.

I was the only one in our group who struck a problem. One of my talks dealt with the care of the very young animal, and this included the care of the pregnant female, the position and development *in utero*, and the birth process. When the school principal learned that I was about to launch upon an unusual and controversial subject he got cold feet, and asked me to check with the local school inspector fifteen miles away. I drove down with some apprehension for inspectors are notorious for their stern manner, and unpliable demeanour. I was therefore very pleasantly surprised when this gentleman gave me a sympathetic hearing which grew into a rehearsal of my entire lecture. Throughout, I had the feeling that this knowledge had been somehow withheld from him all his life, and that he was as eager to assimilate it as the children in my class. "It is certainly time for the young generation to learn that it is not the stork who brings them. Life will be much easier for them than it was for us if they grow into a natural understanding of these matters." He carefully examined the diagram I had brought along; my good friend Angela had made it to demonstrate the position of the foetus *in utero*. Her conception of the subject was exact and informative, a simple black ink drawing on white board. "Carry on, Doctor," the inspector said as I rose to go. "This work is important for our children. I only wish I could be there too."

That year, many children imagined that they wanted to become vets, and I found myself under a barrage of questions and recriminations from some parents. When it was a daughter who expressed the desire to follow my profession, there was a special degree of consternation: some irate mothers came to my door to see what it was all about. "Beg your pardon, Doctor, I know you are a vet, but – well – you are just *different*. We don't want our daughter to become one; if she does no man will ever have her." Some parents craftily let their children come to work with me, for they felt sure that one gruesome operation, one recalcitrant dog, one kick from a horse or one heap of odorous dressings would soon put an end to their ambitions. And so it usually happened; but with a few exceptions, and those were notable.

Among these was a female student, the daughter of a British diplomat, who was doing her schooling in Pretoria. She had travelled extensively and was more mature than most girls of her age. Her mother quietly appealed to me to put her through the hoops and to spare her nothing: her daughter was determined to become a vet, and this summer vacation was her last chance of changing her mind. The fifteen-year-old girl duly arrived, her eyes sparkling with enthusiasm, which was rewarded within the first twenty-four hours: I was called out to attend one of the most appalling cases I have ever seen. On the way there I briefed Helen: "We are going to try and deliver a cow which, the owner admits, has been in labour for four days. Better brace yourself, this is probably going to be a horror of horrors."

It was an unusually hot and sultry day, and the flies were buzzing in their hundreds round the poor beast, which was standing knee-deep in dung and mud. There was no sign of water or fodder; she seemed to balance precariously on her thin legs, forlorn, resigned and heroic as only cows know how to be. We rolled up our slacks, put on rubber aprons, demanded buckets of water and some soap and waded in; we were too stunned by what we saw to remonstrate with the owner, for the time being anyway. The calf had been dead for some time, judging by the process of deterioration it had undergone. I managed to deliver the mangled mass which was impacted in the bovine pelvis; I cleansed the cow internally, treated her with antibiotics to protect the injured tissues from infection, scrubbed up thoroughly and proceeded to give the farmer a piece of my mind. As I spoke I glanced at Helen, standing unruffled in the pungent kraal, and I admired her greatly for her calm manner. If this was her first large-animal case, then she certainly had the makings of a country vet; and I determined to help her get to the veterinary school if I could. That night I sat down to write a letter to her mother. *Your daughter has plenty of spirit and courage – and intelligence. She also has a good sense of humour, which will stand her in very good stead throughout her training and later in practice. I suggest that you confirm her place in the college.* I kept the letter for a week in case something happened to change my mind, but it didn't. Helen grew from strength to strength and seemed to thrive on the more difficult cases. Her one concern seemed to be a fear of missing some decisively horrible case that might settle the matter in her parents' minds.

At last, we were ready to launch into the Bantu school teaching-programme. It had taken some months, but during this time I had gained a great deal of experience, and although I knew that our approach would now be quite different, having been with children and handled their problems helped me enormously. It oiled my mind; I felt it would now be easier to adapt myself to these other children's way of thought. The Bantu children had never had any instruction in animal care or on any subject remotely related to it: we were treading on virgin ground. Power Dzungwe had sent me a formal letter, confirming what he had told me earlier. *Dear Madam*, I read, *I have great pleasure in sending you the names and addresses of the schools in White River area as requested. Some teachers that I talked to about the matter of kindness to animals are very much impressed at this good idea.*

A good idea, but a difficult one to put across. "Kindness to animals" was no obvious matter, when the daily rations which our dogs were receiving in meat alone added up to a week's supply for the average agricultural labourer. In European schools, one could give nutritional advice, one could teach handling and a code of humane behaviour. To gain the confidence of the African child would be a different problem; an African's animals are kept to serve him and sometimes to be his status-symbol too, but their maintenance is usually a matter of the survival of the fittest. Kindness for kindness's sake would mean little at first: we had to approach the subject from another direction.

I was very fortunate in having the help of two friends, both fluent in the various native tongues spoken locally and particularly in Zulu, which is the standard language used in the schools. We spent many evenings in discussion, exploring possibilities: finally we decided to divide the course into three parts, allotting these parts according to our personal inclinations and particular knowledge. The first dealt with folk-lore and the breakdown of superstition, the second with the care of domesticated animals, and the third with practical first-aid, including demonstrations on actual cases.

The naturalist who took the first subject was an expert on African tradition and had grown up among the tribes. He was sensitive and far-sighted, and knew well how gentle he had to be if he was to succeed in this venture. The pointless destruction of owls, chameleons, snakes, porcupines, elephants and many other creatures had always been and still was an accepted everyday occurrence. Tribal law and belief was firmly entrenched: no one could deny that the call of the barn-owl is ghoulish enough to sound like a death-omen, and one can hardly blame the Africans for destroying every one they saw. The tail hair of the elephant was said to give courage and the bones and teeth of certain animals were still used by the witch-doctors. The member of our team who had undertaken this part of the work knew well how deeply embedded in the native mind these beliefs were, and he went about his lectures most circumspectly, explaining the many benefits that man derives from the various animals that he so often kills with no good reason. We had decided to arouse interest by setting essays and drawings on the current subject: these were judged week by week, and prizes were given for the best. The children took to this idea immediately and really enjoyed themselves, giving full vent to their imaginative natures. The results of their enthusiastic labours were a very good yardstick of the impression made upon them, and we were overjoyed to find that their response was far more positive than we had dared to hope.

Here are some of the essays, or parts of them, that were written on two subjects: the breakdown of superstition, and the management of domesticated animals.

The first is by Patrick Dube, fourteen years old, who like most of the Bantu children, began school very late.

> We have a donkey at our home, which we love as if it was a person, because it helps us with many things. We use it to plough mealies, and it also gives manure. When we go to the store to buy goods, we take the donkey to carry them home.
> One day I was herding with my young brother, and we were far from home. It was near a big hill. When we came to this hill it was evening, and when we were starting to go home, my little brother fell from a steep place and broke his leg, and was not able to walk. It was far from home, and I lifted him on to

the donkey which carried him home. When we got there we took him off, and the next morning helped him on again and took him to the doctor at the hospital. Now it seems to me that the donkey is very useful to us natives, who have no cars, bicycles or carts.

(Translated from Zulu.)

Philliman Mdluli wrote the following passages on the bovine:

A Cow

A cow is a domestic animal which has four legs, two horns, two ears, one tail, one head and one udder.

The cow is a helpful animal to everybody. This animal is helpful in many ways. Today we use it for marriage, and it produces perfect food which we call 'milk'. From the milk cream, butter and cheese are made. In summer we use it for ploughing. . . . This animal has been used by the Hottentots. We remember how they bartered their cattle. Most of the wars in the Cape were caused by cattle stealing. This is to show or to prove what a great thing a cow is.

(Written in English. The use of cattle for marriage is a well-accepted custom; the bridegroom pays the bride's father a bride-price in cattle, according to her worth and capabilities as a mother. If she bears no child he demands some of the cattle back.)

An essay by Cathrina Mndaweni, fifteen years old.

The cat is a very useful animal to have in your house because it looks after your possessions. If there are rats it catches them and eats them. Rats eat your clothes and also breed fleas in the house and there are also rats which will gnaw your feet while you are sleeping or will nibble at your hair. . . . If you do not care for your cat well, it will hate you and not stay at home but will go and live in the wild. If you have milk do not withhold it, but give it to the cat, when it will be happy and will like you. Also you must not kill cats, for if you do, when it has done no wrong, you may also die, then you will find the cat in a house in heaven. . . . Your cat is like a lock on your door for it will sit in the doorway and watch the house. It will also make you happy and when it dies, it will remember you, and if you also die you will both meet in heaven. You must remember to do this for we natives often kill cats for no reason, and do not feed them well, as we think that they feed on rats, but we forget that there are days when they do not catch any.

(This little essay (translated) shows how strong is the Bantu belief in the life hereafter. Ancestor-worship is a strong part of their tradition also, but this girl's certainty of the existence of a cat's heaven was very original indeed!)

Victor Sedibe, aged thirteen, wrote a most philosophical little piece, though some of the essence may have been lost in translation:

Tegwane (hammerkop) is useful in keeping down animals, which live in water, for it eats those which bring disease to the water, like mosquitoes and frogs. God gave special work to each kind of animal and Tegwane has also got his work. He kills snakes, mosquitoes, frogs, rats and other small creatures. The tegwane is a bird which eats flesh; another is the owl.

In a similar vein a younger boy, Joseph Madonsela, wrote about birds:

A story about birds

Birds are one of God's creatures, and they are beautiful flying creatures, some birds harmless such as crows, hawk, weaver and guinea-fowls. Birds such as tick-birds are our good friends because they eat ticks on our herds of cattle; birds are not to be killed and chased up and down by us. So they must be freed by us, we must not put them in cages for they help us, by eating insects like borers and caterpillars that destroys our vegetables and our mealie-plants. God has given them wings to fly across the veld and across the rivers, these creatures are clever enough because they can build their nests and feed their youngs without a teacher or being told to do so. Then this must be done by nobody, to take a stone or a gun to kill these poor creatures of God.

(Written in English.)

Lastly, here is an essay written by Samson, who was a very young boy and obviously on the side of the mouse!

Mouse mice

Sometimes at night when it is dark and you are in bed you will hear something scratch, scratch, scratching at the cupboard. What is making that noise? It is a little mouse that is so small that you could hold it in your hand. What was it doing when you heard it scratching with its sharp little teeth, it was trying to bite a hole through hard wood to get some bread that it had smelt with its soft little nose.

(Written in English.)

We were able to judge the progress of our pupils by the many hundreds of such essays we received. Those quoted were all prize-winners; it was a formidable task, each week, to choose which were the best three in each group, for their efforts were quite amazing. While one of us was teaching in one school, another would be starting elsewhere; but often we all went together, one to teach and two to listen for this helped immensely in our assessment of our own work and the children's response to it.

My own classes in practical first-aid also went down well, and in the end the children became very proficient in the various techniques I taught them, such as bandaging, muzzling, extraction of thorns, recognition and basic treatment of snakebite, the administration of medicines, examination of the eyes, ears and body for signs of abnormalities or sickness, the correct way of lifting a pregnant animal and of assistance at birth if necessary, and many other things. I took my own dog along and used him both for demonstration and practice; he very much enjoyed being handled and fondled and fussed over. I also encouraged the children to bring along their own animals, both for the interest of it and so that I could advise them as to treatment if they needed it, which, alas, most of them did. I taught them about traps and snares, pretending that this was new to them, but knowing full well that they were probably adept at all the methods ever devised in this field; for children were often used to set traps while the elders watched from their hiding-places.

It might be optimistic to say that what we taught made a lasting impression; but if this method of teaching was continued and made compulsory, much good would come through it. The teacher's reaction was most gratifying to us, for they said in all sincerity: "Why have we not been told these things before? Will you now come and teach the teachers, so that we can carry on when you have left us?"

My cook and orderly was a wonderful example of a Zulu who, unlike many of his people, showed no fear whatsoever of animals, large or small, with the single exception of the chameleon: he loved working with animals, however fractious they were. Most dogs belonging to white men showed a definite dislike of the black skin, partly through training and partly through instinctive loyalty. It was the same the other way round, and to work with Africans' animals was always difficult for me. Perhaps it was because Sam was fearless that he succeeded so well in handling animals of every description. It is well known that fear produces a subtle secretion, not unlike perspiration, perceptible to animals and specially to those we deem most intelligent, the horse and the dog. My patients responded to Sam's firm touch and gentle manner so wonderfully that many clients remarked upon it, wondering what sort of training he had received. He had received none: no one can teach what Sam already possessed when he came to me.

This was just after our arrival in the White River hills. He came, as so many others did, looking for work, since he and his family were about to be ejected from one of the neighbouring farms. I liked him at once and took him on without further inquiry, and from that time on, for all the years that followed, he worked not so much for us as with us. As his work became more specialised, his status among the surrounding Africans grew, and he was rated as a doctor in his own right. He was humble and self-effacing and very simple, and this position did not seem to go to his head: he continued to live and work as before, while his family lived on the farm at the edge of the plantation in a fine home-made *kaia*.

Once I insulted him, unwittingly, and earned his rebuke. This was at the very beginning: the neighbour's dog had just killed our children's two pet rabbits, and we all ran out to see what all the commotion was about. After the tears and anguish had abated a little, I took the limp bodies and presented them to Sam. "For your wife and children for supper," I said, "I hope they will taste good." The expression on Sam's face was indescribable; horror, contempt, amazement were there, and after a few minutes of silence he quietly handed back the rabbits to me. "Madam", he said with dignity, "I do not eat my friends!"

About that time I became aware that Sam was eating very little meat, no fish and no eggs. I wondered about this, and soon discovered that the reason lay in the teachings of the church which he followed, one of the many local Christian sects. He told me that this, together with teetotalism, also kept him in good health, a very important thing, since he was an ardent soccer player. We often discussed diet, and I found him very sympathetic to my vegetarian way of life; he seemed to understand it much better than most of my white friends.

For a time I employed a young Zulu boy who helped me out in the surgery at the times when I was busiest, our home besieged by an unusual number of visitors and patients, overloading Sam with work. This young boy, Jonah, came from a clerical family and had already decided to follow in his father's footsteps as soon as he could. While driving the long miles to cases we followed a plan of mutual benefit: he would read to me out of the Bible, which he always carried, and I would help him with his English pronunciation; then we would spend some time conversing in Zulu, which I needed very much to improve. On one such morning he began to read a section of the Book of Daniel, with which I was not very familiar.

Suddenly he put down the holy book, gazed at me for some moments and then said with great emphasis: "Doctor, if *you* were thrown to the lions like Daniel, you would not be eaten would you?"

"I hardly think the lions would make an exception of me," I said, very amused, and wondering what train of thought had brought forth this statement.

"Doctor is wrong," he said firmly, "for Doctor is a vegetarian and so was Daniel. The lions would not eat him, therefore they would not touch you either. Now I have read Book of Daniel, I think Doctor very holy!"

I stifled my laughter and turned on the radio, not wishing to discourage his wonderful faith.

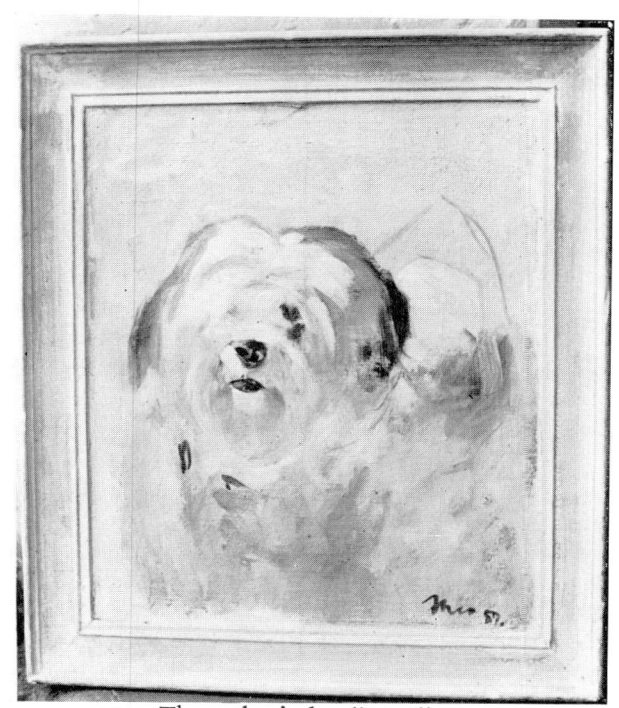

20. The author's dog "Ricci". *From a painting by Theo Papas.*
21. The master potter, Esias Bosch.

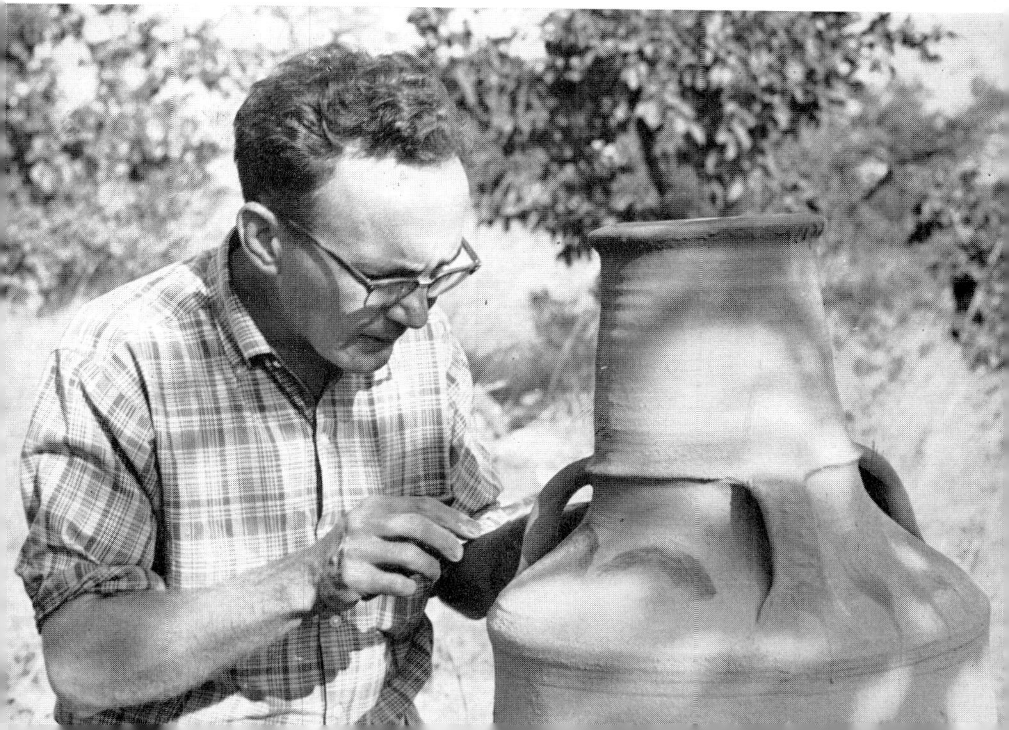

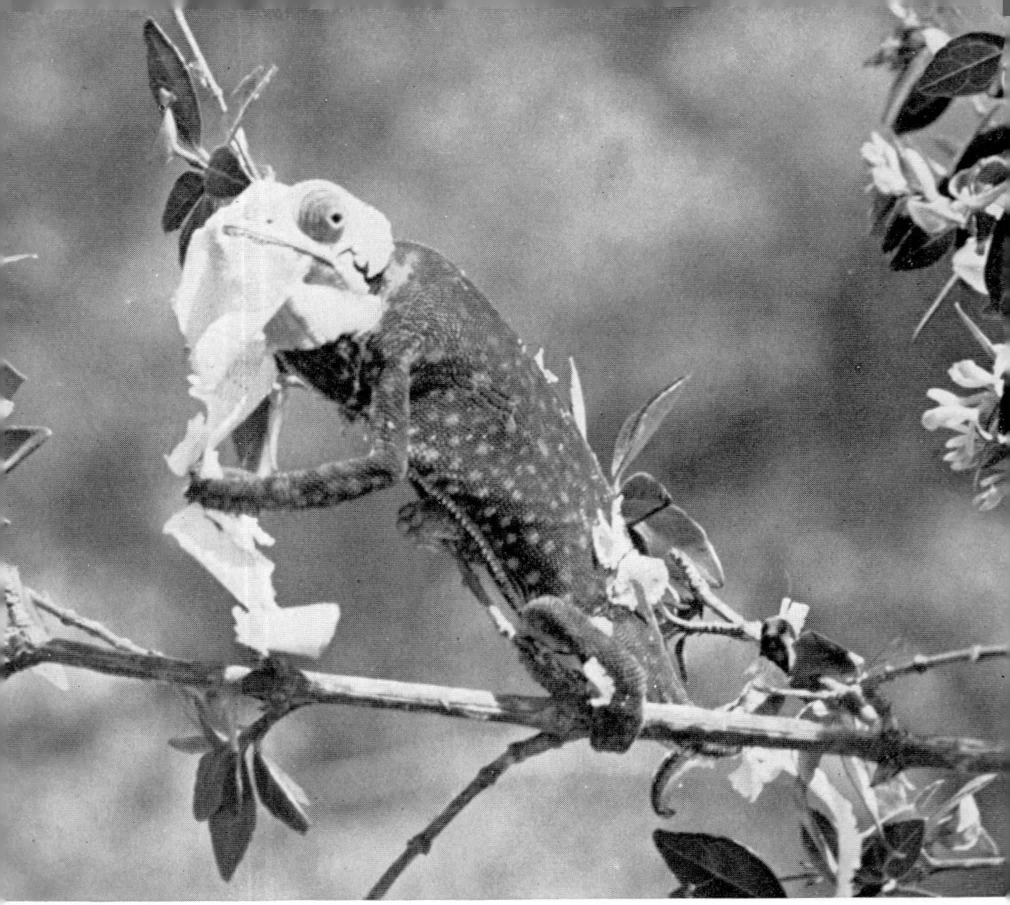

22. Howard Kirk's unique picture of a chameleon stripping off its own skin.
23. Vultures feeding on the remains of a trapped but unclaimed zebra.

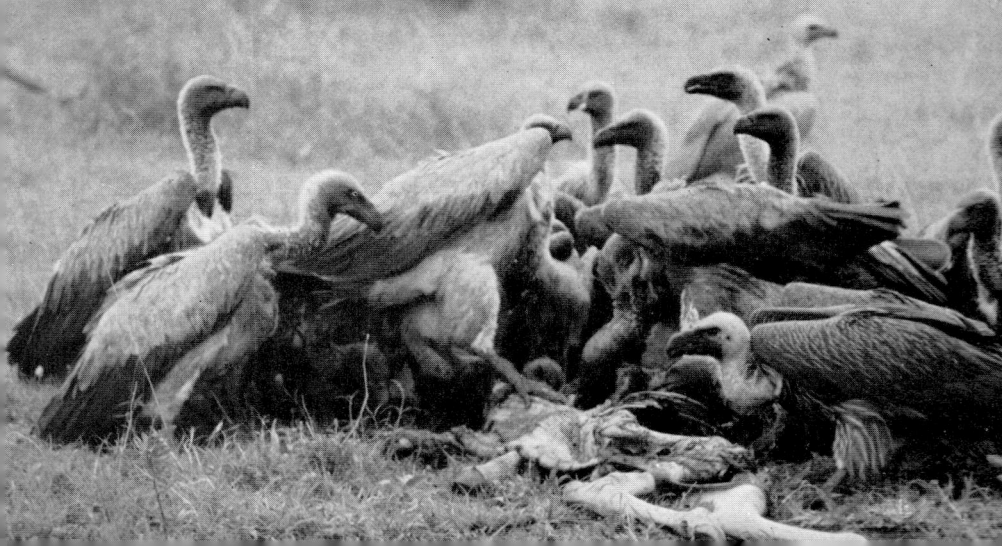

CHAPTER 13

Vultures' Paradise

I had been practising for two years when I began to realise that the most unpleasant aspect of my work – that associated with the treatment of wounds inflicted by man in search of meat – was likely to become closely linked with the most pleasant of all my tasks, that of teaching the young. Only then did this possibility dawn on me: that instead of concentrating upon the adult generation who were inflicting these cruelties, I should rather give my attention to the young. Among all people, whatever their race or creed, it is often the children who teach the grown-ups, influencing them far more than other adults can. In this way my teaching of animal care worked two ways: it impressed children and initiated or fostered their awareness of the animal kingdom, and secondly it helped to bring about a change in the attitude of their parents.

Children are sympathetic and sensitive; they have a streak of cruelty but this can be discouraged when they are very young if more positive thoughts are offered to their very receptive minds. Taught in lively fashion, they always show active and intelligent interest; and their sense of justice can easily be made to override their desire to destroy and to torture, which often arises simply from a need to experiment.

I was very impressed by an incident which occurred about the time I began to teach, and which illustrates this point. A youth, known to be an excellent shot and a great destroyer of wild birds, aimed badly, and a hawk fell to the ground, maimed but not dead. He examined the majestic, limp body and was so overcome with pity and remorse that he implored his father to take him to me, so that I might attempt to heal the bird. He knew how I felt on the subject of bird-shooting, and that he risked a severe reprimand. "Please do something, Doctor Sue," he implored, "I cannot bear to see him like this, bedraggled and suffering." The boy was obviously suffering almost as much as the bird, and he telephoned me at frequent intervals in the days that followed. I performed an operation to remove the pellets which had lodged in the throat, but the hawk died, as I had feared it would, and the boy was inconsolable. He had suddenly entered, with his victim, into the reality of the world of pain; at last he had seen himself as he really was, a wilful poacher on Nature, a butcher of birds. He had no excuse for killing for he was not hungry, nor did he need any part of the bird to ensure his survival. He never shot a bird again, nor did he ever forget that tortured hawk.

Perhaps if it were hunger for meat alone which causes man to poach and to set his deadly traps it would not be so terrible. One can say with truth that in the battle for survival, pain and suffering cannot be avoided; everything must be sacrificed to assuage hunger. Unfortunately it is not like this, except in a few rare cases.

My first introduction to this tragic aspect of life, apart from my contact with domestic pets caught in snares, was when I visited a game farm three hours north, situated on the Olifants river (river of the elephants) in a stretch of country which is distinguished by great scenic beauty. One clear dry morning, while searching for game, we came upon a water-hole situated in the depth of the bush tangle and fed from an underwater spring. The beauty of this drinking-place lay partly in its complete isolation; except for the sound of bird life, an unearthly stillness reigned there. I was most surprised to see two vultures, disturbed by our presence and taking to the air, heavily and reluctantly. The leader of our party froze to attention, listening and sniffing the air as he watched for some moments in absolute silence. This man, whose love and understanding of animal life was so great that he seemed part of that existence more than of ours, had already been responsible for much of my bush education; he had introduced me to the subtleties of the wild, and taught me to look and listen with my eyes and ears fully attentive. Previously I had had no inkling of what may be contained in an apparently immobile and empty corner of wilderness. He gave generously and freely of his self-taught knowledge, so that I also might feel at home in the world he loved.

When I saw him stop so suddenly I knew that there must be something of great interest. Howard moved forward and I followed until we came to the far side of the pool, from which many paths radiated, doubtlessly used by game when coming to drink. We stopped a few yards away from the edge of the little pool, and I saw that I had almost walked into the body of a still living impala (a small buck) ewe which was terribly mutilated, her empty eye-sockets dripping with fresh blood. "This is where the vultures were feeding," said Howard quietly, his jaw muscles clenched tight. "We cannot blame them; eyes are a tasty tit-bit, and it matters little to them whether their victim is alive or dead, providing it keeps still. But look," he added, pointing at the hind leg, "look who is responsible." I had been so mesmerised by the frightful sight that I had not noticed the wire snare, firmly twisted round the upper hind leg, holding the animal fast. It had been dying a slow death from hunger and thirst within sight and smell of grazing and water.

Howard at once delivered the merciful *coup de grace*. When the buck lay quite still at last, he removed the snare and we took it with us, as evidence both for the owner of the farm and for reference later on when we were teaching in schools. As we moved away we were almost caught by a thick cable loop which dangled from a branch, obviously intended for larger game such as zebra or giraffe. From here our party split up and we searched the whole area within a quarter of a mile. Between us we found sixteen snares of various sizes. Some of the wires still held putrefying flesh; one thick noose gripped the long leg-bone of a giraffe, which had doubtlessly died and been consumed by hyenas or other scavengers. The bone was grooved by the animal's struggles before it died.

That day, the needless suffering and despair of these snared creatures was brought home to me as never before. My interest grew, and I devoted time to learning more about this underworld of pain for which man is responsible.

It appears that within the Republic of South Africa, where the Bantu are not permitted to carry firearms, the wire snare, which is easily obtainable, provides a cheap means of killing animals. Steel cables – made as brake-cables for cars – are most often used, and they are sold for this purpose by unscrupulous storekeepers.

Single-stranded wire, such as baling wire, is used for smaller animals, but it is more wasteful, since it sometimes gives way under strain: then the animal breaks away with a tight ring of wire round the neck or limb. I have never forgotten the sight of the huge majestic elephant in Mozambique, blowing sand over his ensnared leg which was still trailing the cable, no doubt to cool it and lessen the pain. He would probably continue to live for some time in an agonised state until he succumbed to general septicaemia. I have also seen elephant with most of their trunk missing, victims of the same method, and these would try to feed while kneeling – a hopeless process, ending with emaciation and death.

Snares and traps are set in a number of different ways; the simplest consists of placing a large number wherever there are suitable gaps in the vegetation, or on paths used by animals. As this method is rather haphazard, the snares have to be left for long periods before a visit by the trappers becomes worth while. This method is also the one used for choice at drinking places. The poacher's task here is much easier, and sometimes every possible approach to the water is set with traps. Sometimes these are actually set underneath the surface of the water, attached to logs of wood: they may catch wildebeest or zebra, which crowd the waterholes in the dry season.

Where these methods are not suitable because of the vegetation, branches are laid across the animals' probable line of movement. Gaps are left at intervals and in each of these a snare is set. Operating in gangs and mostly at night, the poachers first locate a herd and then, using a barrier, they drive the game into it with dogs. These dogs are well trained and give the alarm at the approach of strangers; this makes it difficult for patrols to arrest anyone, even if they have a good idea where the poaching party is operating. To make arrest less likely the gangs do not, as a rule, stay in one area for more than one night.

Another atrocious method of trapping makes use of a sapling, which is pegged down and has a wire noose attached. When an animal moves into this snare, the pressure is released and the animal is pulled upwards, where it remains suspended until it is killed by the poachers or else dies of its injuries, hunger and thirst. Monkeys are often caught in this way for sale as pets. As this work is very hurried, a number of animals often break away, sometimes with snares attached; many empty snares are left behind as there is not always time to collect them. The game meat is used mainly for making biltong (dried meat, cut into strips) and this finds a ready sale among the Bantu in town and country areas as well as in the native reserves.

The most tragic aspect of this, apart from the suffering caused to individual animals, is the fact that the native people make use of only an extremely small proportion of the animals killed. Apart from the use of fire for driving game, this must be one of the most wasteful methods of killing ever devised. The poachers cannot visit the snares regularly, least of all when they are set at random in the bush. As a result of this, large numbers of the animals caught are devoured by scavengers, or decay before they can be claimed. This is especially true of the smaller animals, such as impala, which may be devoured by vultures in a matter of minutes and at night are eaten by hyenas. It is seldom, indeed, that such an animal is taken as an intact carcase.

In the case of large animals, such as giraffe, there is also a great deal of waste, as poachers are unable to take away more than a small portion of the meat for fear of detection. Few animals manage to free themselves from the noose, but a very considerable number manage to break the wire. When this happens the loop is usually left intact on the victim, which, through its struggles, has drawn it extremely tight; animals have been found with such circlets cutting the jaws, head, neck, base of horn, and limbs. As can be imagined, the cutting effect of the wire usually leads to the eventual death of the animal; and the manner of his death may be slow and protracted.

It seems clear that for every animal claimed by the poacher a large number are wasted. It is not an exaggeration to say that poachers are lucky to find the carcase of one in ten animals killed in snares. Trophy hunters, too, are a terrible curse in Africa, for they will kill a lion for no other reason than to get his feet for their tribal ceremonies, or chop off the tail of a wildebeest to be used as a decoration and a fly-switch.

The Africans are not by any means the only ones guilty of poaching. Europeans use firearms for this sport, working on foot or from vehicles with the help of spotlights. In the glare, the eyes of the hunted beast are seen easily; but this is a most wasteful method, since it is extremely difficult to find a wounded animal at night. It has often amazed me that people, who to my certain knowledge are guilty of killing illegally (though I have lacked the proof to prosecute) may also become genuinely concerned and even outraged when their own pet comes home dragging a wire snare. They are much more to blame than the Africans whom they loudly abuse for setting traps: the latter have at least a tradition of hunting for survival, while the white man poaches only because he is unwilling to pay for a hunting licence, or else because he likes to eat cheap meat himself and feed it to his labour force.

In veterinary practice, trap wounds are a common occurrence. On an average, every third animal caught in a snare returns home mostly mutilated and sometimes in the last stage of exhaustion, reaching its doorstep with the last breath before total collapse. The deadly 'gin' trap takes the greatest toll, for it is impossible for a trapped animal to free itself from this cruel, cumbersome, and heavy piece of bare-toothed metal. I have known animals to return home after a week in such a trap, having torn away the macerated limb in one last, courageous effort to save themselves. Sometimes a wire loop catches the animal round the throat. This happened in the case of an adult male cat which I was called to see just in the nick of time, for it was at the point of strangulation. The owner did not know that the cat had been snared and was alarmed when he came home, breathing with difficulty, the neck and head swollen and the tongue slightly protruding and blue. I placed my fingers round the neck and became aware of a tight constriction, discovering at the last moment that a fine wire was deeply embedded round the throat. We found some wire cutters and managed to remove the snare, and were rewarded greatly by the immediate relief to the cat.

This wire noose was very useful to me in the next talks I gave, in African and European schools alike. Living examples were important, children are always far more impressed by particular cases than by routine instruction and generalisation. I took particular care to keep very detailed case accounts from this time on; unfortunately I was never short of material of this sort, for week after week some animal would be brought in, buck or bird, dog or cat. To teach children about the evil of trapping and poaching was a long-term policy; given time and the wide use of similar methods, some success may be achieved. I can see no other way of ensuring the preservation of wild life in the future.

CHAPTER 14

Gonzo the Giant

My new experiences in schools gave me not only a better understanding of children's relationships with animals, but also a greater insight into the psychology of my own patients; and of their owners as well. Animals, I discovered, behaved quite differently with and without their masters and mistresses, and differed immensely in their ability to endure pain, their impatience, their intelligence, just as humans do. I found myself observing them more closely and wishing that I could devote another lifetime to studying animal psychology. The opportunities of a veterinarian to study this field are unique, for the real personality of a dog or cat is displayed far more vividly under adverse circumstances or stress. Observation takes time, however, and unless the patients were taken in for a lengthy period the conclusions drawn would be incomplete, though very interesting.

Among dogs there is an immense variety of behaviour patterns. Environment, upbringing, occupation in the case of working dogs, heredity – these all play vital parts in the formation of their characters. They are blessed and cursed with virtues and vices just as we are. They can be moody, sympathetic, self-pitying, loyal, heroic, cowardly; and their traits are as varied as their physical characteristics. The dog does not attempt to mask or disguise his character; he does not pretend to be joyful when sad because he thinks he should, nor does he try to control his temper when he is angry. Even though he lives such an uninhibited life, he still gets duodenal ulcers; and lung cancer as well, though he doesn't smoke. No two dogs seem to be alike, yet they all have one thing in common; their love for their master is unconditional. Whatever his mood, their tails (if they have any) are wagging and their ears are pricked for a word of affection. When a dog dies and is replaced by another, although the one may have been a poodle and the other a Great Dane, there is one common character which is present in all canines, an intangible quality which shines through and which makes the grief one feels at a loyal friend's departure, so much the less. There are very few dogs which are spontaneously mean and revengeful; an uneven temperament is usually the result of wrong handling and human neurosis. Yet I have occasionally met dogs which are unfriendly, even though the owners were kind and thoughtful people. Perhaps their prenatal experiences were unfavourable!

The ability to endure pain does not vary from breed to breed, as is often thought, but from individual to individual. There are certain breed-characteristics which are obvious, as obvious as the physical weaknesses which often result from inbreeding — the spine of the dachshund, the urinary composition of the Dalmatian, the dermoid cyst of the Rhodesian ridgeback. Two contrasting dogs were once brought in to me at the same time, contrasting both in character and in physical appearance. Both came to stay for one month and both were to have surgical treatment. The older of the two was a Great Dane dog, a massive dog weighing about 140 lbs. The younger was a black poodle female weighing nine pounds. They were so completely different that they hardly seemed to belong to the same species at all; yet from the first moment of their meeting they became the closest friends, which made their stay all the more enjoyable, for them and for us.

Gonzo, the big Great Dane, was the epitome of the handsome Prince Charming; he stole Gigi's heart, and it seemed that he was as enamoured of her diminutive shape as she was of his vast, smooth-skinned, honey-coloured bulk. They sat in my waiting-room together and eyed each other calmly; he was quiet, genteel, noble, generous, in fact the perfect gentleman; she was feminine and helpless in the extreme and no doubt irresistible, for her noisy and somewhat neurotic nature might otherwise have frightened the Dane away. She was highly intelligent and imaginative, he less clever and more realistic. "Thank goodness I have *you* to look after me," I could almost hear her say as she gazed at him appealingly over the decorated leash; "if you weren't there I would just fall to pieces!" It is hard to imagine how she would have behaved if he had, indeed, not been there to give moral support; as it was, her conduct was a great trial to all of us.

Gonzo had caught his right fore-leg in a gin-trap; he was

missing for a week before his master discovered him, many miles from home and in a pitiable state. He was emaciated and burning with fever, the stench of putrefying tissues detectable even through the mountain of bandages and disinfectant that had been applied. Without a moment's hesitation, he leapt upon my high examination table when his master quietly ordered him to do so, shook hands with me after lying down on command, and allowed himself to be handled without a murmur, though his wincing eyes told a different story. Afterwards he licked my hand with a touching gesture of spontaneous gratitude. When his owners drove away he looked longingly after them for a moment, his ears drooping; but when I approached him a few moments later to put on his chain, he wagged his tail and put on a brave face, allowing himself to be led into the sick-bay without resistance – stoical, optimistic and trusting. Only when he lay down on his mattress did he heave a great sigh, his whole body seeming to tremble with sadness.

Gigi had come for pre-operative treatment of enlarged, chronically infected tonsils; she was to have a tonsillectomy as soon as her enlarged glands regressed. It was impossible to handle her in the presence of the owner, and even without her it took at least two of us to hold Gigi still so that her throat could be examined. Her slippery, agile little body was far more difficult to handle than that of her heavy-muscled friend, and my heart sank at the thought that she would be with us for thirty whole days.

When I realised, simply from their behaviour on meeting in my waiting-room, that the two dogs had something in common, I decided to kennel them together for an initial period at least. Gonzo rose politely as I entered with the poodle, and seemed extremely pleased to welcome her into his lair. It is always good therapy to house two patients together when this is feasible, for loneliness and boredom can retard healing. The dogs looked at each other and sniffed as was their custom, Gonzo deferentially and Gigi in unashamedly aggressive fashion after which they seemed to reach a mute understanding and settled down to enjoy their newfound companionship.

By the time Gigi's tonsils had regressed, Gonzo's temperature had dropped sufficiently for me to attempt amputation. I prepared him in other ways in order to strengthen him, and as his appetite was poor, I had to use other than oral means. Their operations were planned for the same morning, and both were successful. Within three days Gonzo, though heavy and by no means young, had partly rehabilitated himself and was able to move freely on three legs. He was obviously proud of his achievement and a new note crept into his interesting character: he had previously appeared modest and quiet, but now he performed all sorts of tricks to gain our attention. He seemed happiest when the time came each morning to change his dressings, and his heroism was amazing to witness, for it is well known from human patients that an amputated stump is very painful indeed. His behaviour remained constant at those times; he would leap on to the table, lie down, wag his tail as though to tell me that he was ready, lick my hand, and quietly wait for me to begin. He winced occasionally, sometimes even a whine would escape from his lips, but he always cancelled it out with a tail-wag when I had finished the painful task of dressing the new raw stump. He would then give me another lick and jump down from the table. Sometimes he would hang his long-eared head over the edge of the table and literally smile at Gigi, reassuringly, and then she would cease to moan in anticipation, though she knew well that her turn came next. Her behaviour was entirely different from his: she would do anything to escape attention, and would hide in the most impossible places whenever the time came to give her post-operative care.

I often tried to trick her. By this time, both dogs were living in the house with the rest of our vast menagerie, which included two bush babies, guinea-pigs, dogs, cats, various birds, bovines and equines. When I entered the room where Gigi was, if my intentions were 'honourable' she would welcome me and leap on to my lap without hesitation. But if I so much as allowed a cunning thought to cross my mind, if I pretended to be sociable when I merely wanted to find a way to capture her, she would sense it immediately and retreat under the settee, from which sanctuary it was difficult to unearth her. Often she would run to Gonzo for moral support, if he was near by, and hide behind him. He would look at me apologetically with his limpid brown eyes, as if to say: "you must excuse her, she is so fragile and helpless!"

Unfortunately the children noticed at once that she resembled a certain lady very closely, and insisted on calling her Mrs. P. from the first. As chance would have it, this same person called on me in connection with some charitable work she hoped I would do for her organisation, though I had been trying to avoid this for some time. As we were having a cup of tea we were startled by my little son Guy rushing into the lounge and announcing that Mrs. P. had just made a puddle on the best Persian rug. "She's done it again!" he said, and then he spotted our visitor and reversed out of the room with lightning speed, mumbling something about wiping it up before the dark spot became too big. Mrs. P. rose stiffly from her seat and prepared to leave, and as she did so almost fell over her canine counterpart, who had fled from the loud recriminations of my son. When Gigi felt the heavy heel of the insulted lady, she began to vocalise loudly, in more or less the same tone of voice which our visitor used, thus adding vocal resemblance to physical likeness and suggesting that the two had been cast in the same mould, though their earthly form differed somewhat. I had stumbled upon a useful method of avoiding unwelcome activities!

I have often wondered whether a dog and his owner actually grow to resemble each other. Is it perhaps just a case of buying a breed of dog which resembles oneself? If so, the intention is probably subconscious! Does man, or woman grow like dog, or does dog grow like man? If personalities merge, then the process should be gradual; which perhaps it is. It is often the aggressive man who owns a fox-terrier, the heavy-built short-breathed man who buys a bulldog; the sleek, well-groomed man owns a black labrador (and a long low black car with purple upholstery) while the short, stout, busy housewife keeps a pug.

To quote an extreme case: the borzoi, which was originally imported from Russia, gives the impression of having been literally flattened in a clothes-mangle. To suggest that a person could resemble such a shape may seem far-fetched, yet much of what a vet sees in the course of practice borders on fantasy in any case. The owner of such a borzoi, Christopher Henkel, seemed entirely like his dog from the head downwards: his pointed nose, his slanting eyes, his benevolent personality. When they came in to me and stood in the doorway together, the likeness was so strong as to be ridiculous; if one day the dog had arrived leading his long, lean master, I would hardly have noticed the difference.

Another example of this type of family resemblance was that between an old, much-loved resident of the Lowveld, Andrew Rusk, whose face, accent and personality were thoroughly Scottish, and his big yellow cross-bred bull-mastiff dog. They were uncannily alike; even their mannerisms seemed similar. They both tilted their heads in exactly the same welcoming manner; they sat erect and proud, side by side in the car as they sped by. The dog did not actually bark with a Scottish brogue as did his master, but we took it for granted that had he ever broken into English, it would have been in the manner of his master, Andrew.

There are those who live for their dogs. This type of relationship can lead to much heartache, for in the end comes the inevitable parting, bringing sorrow to the survivor, though it is not necessarily a human survivor who suffers most. I am privileged to have known such a twosome, though in this case they were permitted to leave this earth within a few hours of each other. The man was very old and very frail, a widower. His collie dog was equally ancient, if one applied the standard of age set by man for the canine – one human year equal to seven canine years. The old man had been ailing for a very long time and his affliction was severe and of a wasting nature. He refused to see a doctor, and he always told me, when I attended his dog, that his great aim in life was to pass away with his beloved dog, which, I suspected, was suffering from abdominal cancer. The welfare of this man lay heavily upon my conscience, for it seemed clear that as long as I could keep his dog alive he would survive also. I visited the pair each week, and each time the condition of each had worsened. Yet in the poverty and the distress of that little household there was something which filled me with warmth and optimism. The devotion and love of this pair for each other was perhaps the most touching thing I have ever witnessed. They were enough for each other, and content to wait without fear; it should have been terrible to go into that gloomy shack, but it was wonderful, and very humiliating. They finally died, within a few hours of each other, when I had gone on leave; the old man's daughter, who was visiting him at the time, told me of it.

A week after my return I was asked to give a talk to a local society. I decided to break away from the usual topics upon which every vet holds forth at some time or other. 'Preventive Medicine', or 'Diseases of Animals Communicable to Man', or 'Why and How I Became a Vet': I had worn a groove into these subjects, and I wanted to get away from them.

"What will be your subject this time?" asked the president of the society. "I just want to know so that I can announce it."

"It will be about the similarity between dogs and their owners," I answered rashly, and was amused to see that my friend had not taken me seriously.

"Never mind, we know what a busy person you are. Let me know later."

That night I thought about the problem very deeply; and as usual I consulted my friend, Athalie Waugh, whose opinion I valued highly and who was the most outspokenly honest person I have ever met. "Do you think people mind knowing that their neuroses are transmitted to their dogs?" I asked her on the phone. "I feel it's about time the locals saw themselves as they are! – though I would try to be tactful." I explained the situation to her, and as I did so her inimitable humour overcame her and she burst into peals of unrestrained laughter. There was an ominous click somewhere on the party line.

"Someone listening in again," she said, "let's give them their money's worth!" And she proceeded, in a manner which was really worthy of her, to throw a few comparisons down the party-line which must have made a deep impression! "I think it is a wonderful idea," she chuckled, "you go ahead, but leave me out of it."

"You'd come out of it very well," I answered, "if I compared you with your silver-coated ghosts. Nothing neurotic in your family, even your parrot is normal. I'd have to give up practice if everyone was like you."

"Don't speak too soon," she said; and indeed, one week later, her beautiful grey dog was dead with snake-bite. She died as I opened my medical case, victim of a rhinghals.

So I took my courage into both hands, and on the appointed day gave an address on the subject of the pet-owner relationship. I gave many examples; I spoke of the restless, the unhappy, the over-possessive and the overwrought, and explained how these mental states played a vital part in the disease syndrome. I told them that an owner, who is out of balance on those lines can not only cause physical sickness in himself, but also transmit his unhappiness and his tensions to his pet. I tried hard to stay away from too many obvious local comparisons, but I know that many felt implicated that day and smiled and said nothing. "Children are exactly the same," I added in conclusion. "Their existence is closely tied up with their parents' emotions. Their health will suffer if you are unhappy, and in the extreme their mental balance will suffer too. The power we wield over our dependants is enormous, and hence our responsibility is the greater."

I was introduced to this train of thought when I was still a student. I was practising in London, or rather assisting in a practice, when a pekingese dog was brought in by a well cciffured and beautifully dressed woman. The dog was very ill – dehydrated, distressed, vomiting at regular intervals, his coat dry and his skin tight. I happened to be on duty and I examined the dog minutely, but could find nothing wrong with him at all which could have given rise to such serious symptoms. Not wishing to seem too inexperienced I suggested that the dog be taken in for observation for one week. This was agreed upon, and by the next day the dog already appeared brighter, though he had received no treatment and had not eaten. His improvement continued, and by the end of the week he was feeding normally and appeared glossy and bright. The owner took him home most gratefully and praised me effusively, which was somewhat embarrassing as I had done nothing at all for the dog except confine him. Within five days the little peke was back again with the same symptoms, the owner suggesting that he must have suffered a relapse. By now the other members of the practice had become interested, and we watched and examined him carefully each day for the following week. There was no sign of disease; the dog, we concluded, was under mental stress and this was sufficient to produce those extensive symptoms. I wondered what turmoil lay beneath the well-rouged face of his mistress, and how best to suggest that she should part with her dog. I left this to the seniors and never knew how they managed it so tactfully; in the end she sold the dog, and phoned me to thank me for all my loving care.

The sensitivity of dogs varies as much as do their other characteristics. There is the insensitive hound who just plods along from day to day and is little affected by a change which will send the next dog almost mad with fright and apprehension. The sensitive dog is affected by anything from humidity to electric charges and astral entities. I had often heard it said that dogs can see ghosts, but I hardly believed it, perhaps because in those days I did not, or dared not, believe in ghosts myself. The first time I had evidence of this super-sensitiveness of the dog was at one of the showplaces of the Lowveld, one of its breathtaking beauty-spots whose surroundings, even to the seasoned world-traveller, are unique. To the east lies the country of Mozambique and the coastal region ; to the north lies the 'sea' of bushveld, the Kruger National Park beyond, the areas of the native reserves, hazy with dust and heat, domain of wild game and haven of the poacher. To the west lie the mountains of the Sabie Valley up to the jagged blue heights of Maryps kop, contrasting strongly with the more distinctively African scenery which lies thirty miles away. To the south are the gentle hills and pine-forests of the farming areas, sloping into the gums and subtropical plantations which are the source of local wealth.

The lawns surrounding the homestead had been mown to a smooth green carpet and were fringed with lilies and flaming red Christ's Thorn and tropical shrubs. The bamboos towered above, creaking and swaying in the almost constant refreshing breeze that makes this climate almost alpine and temperate. A mission-house had been beautifully and artistically converted into a stately home, inhabited now by two people strange and unusual as well as very artistic. In their home I felt a mixture of fascination and repulsion, as did many others who visited it, and each time I drove away I felt certain that here a strange influence was at work, though I could not define it.

Very early one morning I passed the entrance drive after I had made a call in that direction; and I felt impelled to turn back a little, so that I could spend a few moments with my unusual friends. They were not in, and so I decided to take a few minutes' break on their lawn and drink my fill of their view. I heard soft padding footsteps behind me, and I turned, startled; here, anything could happen, and I was always on the alert. Then I saw the dog, the only one who had stayed there for any length of time: a long-haired cross, large and rough, breed unknown. He came

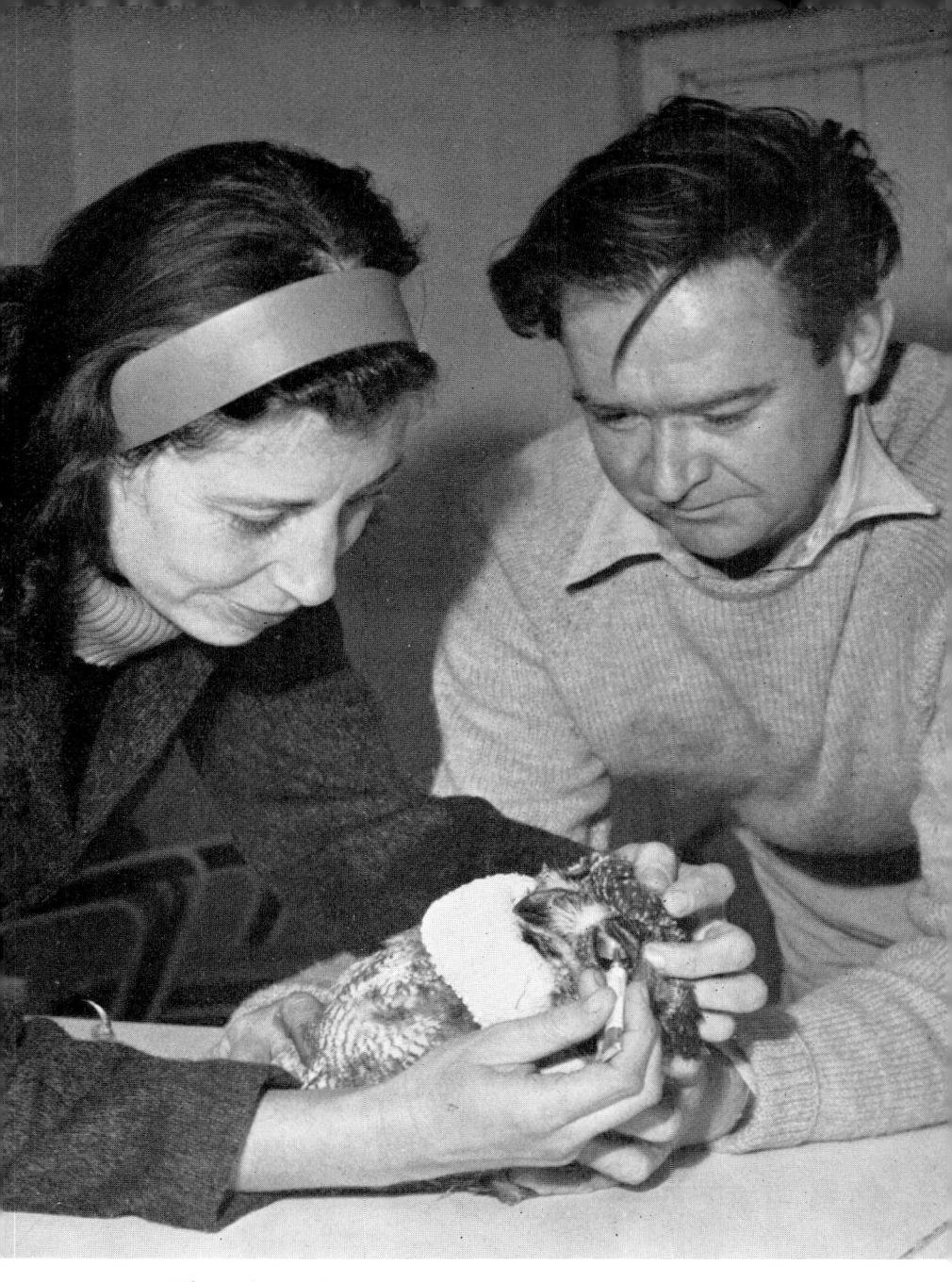
24. The author and Howard Kirk treating an owl for an injured eye.

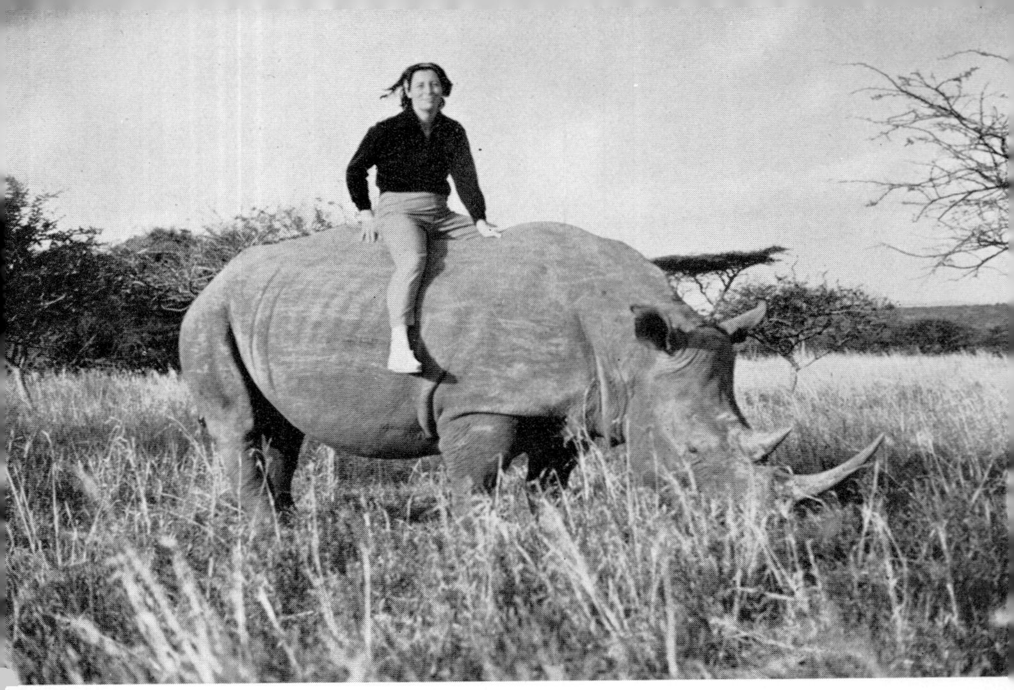

25. "I was looking far from confident." The author astride a wild white rhino.

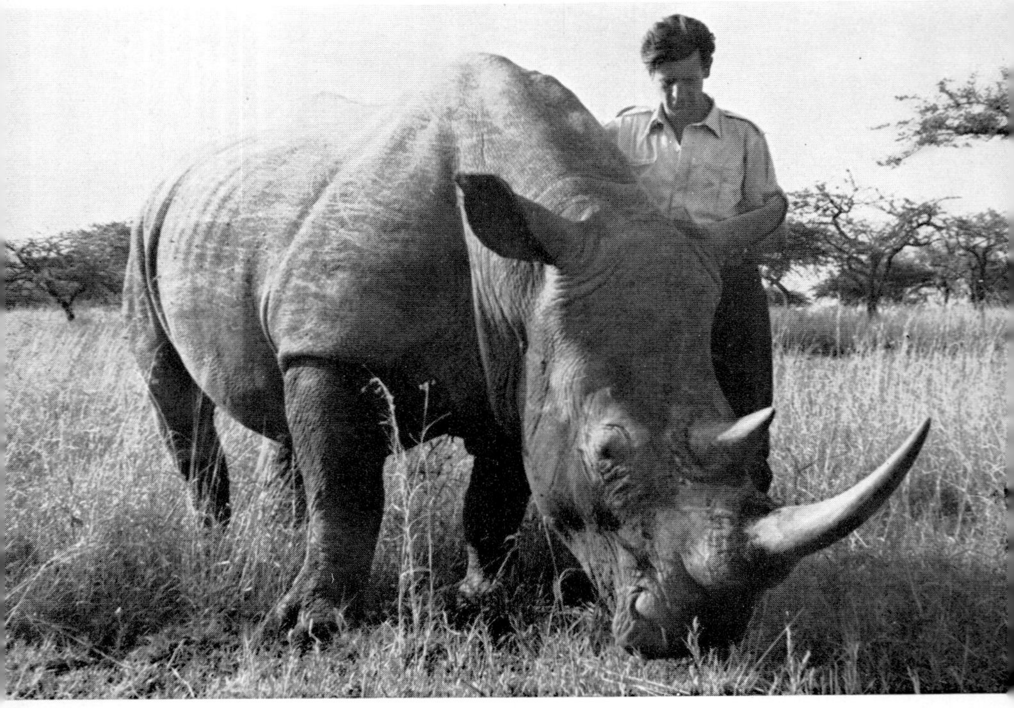

26. John Clarke with one of his beloved white rhinos.

towards me with his tail wagging, eager for company. As I touched his coat I saw that his yellow eyes suddenly opened wide, staring beyond me towards the banana hills. I saw his hackles go up and his body twist away from me in one movement. There must have been something there, but I could not see it; I seemed to sense another presence, but later told myself that this could only have been imagination – I was already in that frame of mind. The dog broke away from my grip and backed away, eyes agape, tail and ears down, seeing a world beyond me into which I could not follow. Before he disappeared from view he gave a blood-curdling howl which brought me staggering to my feet and sent me racing for my station-wagon, parked beyond the blazing thorns. I tried to sort out my thoughts on the way back but could not; the only thing I knew for certain was that the dog had seen an astral entity.

This incident proved very helpful to me a little later on, when I was called to see a very distressed family whose dog was troubling them past the limit of patience. The lady of the house was a delightful and balanced person, and I had known her for some time. She told me that recently, at the same hour each day, her dog had become restless, rushing from person to person in an effort to gain attention and – even more curiously – seeming to ask for protection. Just before sunset, after about an hour of this strange display, the dog became calm again, and behaved as though nothing unusual had happened. I went along one afternoon later to witness the dog's antics, and examined him in the surgery the next day. He seemed in excellent health and so I suggested that he should stay with me, and that I would watch him carefully at the time before sunset.

The experiment proved that whatever troubled him did not exist in my home. To make sure, I kept him for three days, with the same results. Then I took him back with some sedatives, and instructed the owner to let me know how he was within five days. She could not wait so long, and telephoned me in two days to say that he was still having his "drink-time jitters" and would I please come up again, for this was getting beyond endurance. That evening I watched him intently as he worked himself into a frenzy, when it suddenly occurred to me that there was something familiar about the look of him, especially his eyes. He seemed to be looking beyond us, and then rushing back to ask protection from his mistress. "I've got it." I jumped up, and in my eagerness my client almost dropped her glass with fright. "He is seeing a ghost! A clairvoyant would confirm it." Darkness was falling, and with it relaxation and quiet came to the dog, which curled up on the rug, exhausted. "Has anyone died recently in your family?" I asked, expecting to be ridiculed for my suggestion. There was a long silence. "You may be right," the lady said, "someone did die here a little while ago, and the dog was very much attached to her. This is the only explanation that makes sense."

And so the riddle was solved. After four months the restless spirit left, and the dog ceased his jitters. By common agreement the whole episode was kept discreetly quiet: who would wish to publicise the fact that they had a family ghost?

CHAPTER 15

Ride a Wild Rhino

Whenever during my years of veterinary practice I have enjoyed an unusual run of success and have mentally patted myself on the back, some disaster has invariably occurred and brought me back to earth very smartly. "We are not permitted to savour our successes," a good friend once told me from his own bitter experience, "success is always succeeded by failure!"

After the episode of the haunted dog, I felt that I had really made some progress in my understanding of canine psychology. I was just writing up the case-history when my faithful Sam came in to tell me that he was having trouble with one of the cats. "Time for big black cat to go home," he said meaningfully, "she terrible nuisance, she tried to bite me, and her teeth opened my skin." (In spite of the fact that this happened to be a male cat, Sam always insisted in calling all felines female, just as he called all canines male.) I examined the wound and dressed it, small though it was, for cat bites are most unpleasant and usually turn septic. "All right, then, let us put him in a basket and I will take him home." We picked up a basket from the cattery and advanced upon the cage, armoured with gloves. The cat must have seen us coming, for he was ready, and as we carefully opened the door he sprang at us, teeth bared and claws extended: in our surprise we could not hold him for more than a moment. As I tried to stop him, he twisted out of my grip and escaped into the long grass, disappearing from view with great speed. "She is running home," Sam shouted at me and he tried to follow, "I think we lose her now." Which indeed we had, and I cursed myself for feeding the black terror so well: a leaner cat would have been less adventurous. There was no sign of him as we ran down to the end of the farm, for he was wary and intelligent, and determined that we should not lay our hands on him again and repeat his sufferings.

It was no use putting it off – I had to telephone the owner

immediately, for nothing is more embarrassing than a patient reaching its home unexpectedly! "Hello, Mrs. Rowe, how are you?" I began with hesitation, "I've phoned to tell you about your cat."

"How very kind of you, dear Doctor Sue, I was just thinking of my precious Fluff; I miss him so much. Is he ready to come home yet?"

"He is on his way now, should reach you in anything from three hours to three days."

The dear lady laughed like a bell. "Oh, you are so funny, Doctor. Such a lovely sense of humour. Wonderful how you keep so jolly when you are so busy!"

"I am afraid I am in deadly earnest, Mrs. Rowe; your cat is so well that he would not allow himself to be confined any longer, and decided to go home to his beloved mistress all by himself this morning. I am very sorry about it."

There was a lengthy silence, "Ooooh."

My heart was beating at double speed, and although I kept telling myself that the welfare of one terrible black cat could not possibly weigh on my conscience, somehow I could not really convince myself of the truth of this. From the very beginning it had been drummed into us that the worst disgrace a vet can incur is to let a patient escape. It doesn't matter whether it is a pet mouse or a horse, it just doesn't pay to be careless – for one escape can ruin one's reputation overnight. Yet, inevitably, once or twice in every vet's life this does happen; and for once one is completely thrown on the mercy of the client, for the making or breaking of one's professional good name.

"Poor Doctor!" came the unexpected exclamation across the wires, startling me out of my apprehensive reverie, "I am sorry for you. Don't worry too much; he will find his way sooner or later, and I will let you know just as soon as he does. We'll keep this our little secret, won't we? Other people might take it the wrong way, and say it was due to your carelessness. But I know better; my little Fluff just loves me so much that nothing would keep him away. Bye now, have a nice day!" Had Mrs. Rowe not been separated from me by the telephone, I would have thrown my arms around her and kissed her, so great was my relief. "A client will always turn on you and give you away," my professor had once said; and to find one soul who did the opposite, restored a great deal of my faith in human nature. After two days this lady phoned me to say that Fluff had indeed returned to her, a little burr-covered, but otherwise none the worse for wear. "Should I bring him back to you for a check-up, my dear?" she asked. My heart sank: I just couldn't face this all over again! "I'll come and see him at your house when I pass tomorrow, just to check the operation site. Meanwhile keep him quiet, and thank you so much for putting my mind at rest."

I was very fortunate to get off so lightly, for on a previous occasion I had really lost a dog just after a major operation. This was terrible: the little fox-terrier was asleep on the floor of the car one moment, and in the next – while I went into the house, leaving the door ajar – she disappeared completely and utterly without trace. How a dog could suddenly recover from Pentothal anaesthesia sufficiently to go romping off into the fields, especially with a long, new abdominal wound, was a puzzle I never solved, I could only think of my own appendectomy, one year before. after which I suffered more pain and discomfort than I had imagined possible, finding it difficult to leave the bed after forty-eight hours to take even a few steps.

We searched endlessly, informing all the neighbours, but were finally forced to inform the owners, the police and the local S.P.C.A. When after twelve hours there was still no news I could only assume the worst, and my clients were at the end of their tether. It was bad enough trying to imagine what the little dog was going through, if she still lived, but perhaps her owners' distress was even greater. The dog was old and very frail, and as each hour passed my client's reproach grew stronger and my own shame deeper.

That evening after the search had been abandoned, I received a visit from the headmaster of the local Bantu school, a delightful, well-educated and very humble man. "I will not trouble you for long, Doctor," he said, "for I have lessons to prepare for tomorrow. I have come first to inquire how is Doctor's health, for I hear she has been ill with the flu." We exchanged family news, and I discovered that his valiant wife had just borne another baby. He confided that it was a boy-child and not a 'no-good' girl, and that he was happy to think that he now had three boys who would take care of them in his old age. Then we discussed the new programme for teaching in African schools; he had helped me well with this and given me much-needed encouragement at the beginning, when I had not been at all sure how to tackle such a project. (It had also been he who had welcomed me on to the farm when I had first come to the Lowveld, some years before; he came to represent his community, giving me a touching welcome, the sort of welcome which everyone needs when entering a new country and a new venture. He came, formally dressed in a suit, on his bicycle, with his wife beside him, flanked by several children, all immaculately dressed. He stood in the back garden, chatting to Sam until I came out to see who was there. He then assumed a formal stance, put back his shoulders, and gave a charming speech of welcome, expressing, as he said, the feeling of all his people. "We welcome you with all our heart, doctor of animals, and we hope to have you here for many years to come. May our cows and donkeys bear many babies under your care and may you yourself bear many too. Please come for any help if you need it." He then presented his wife, a robust, sweet-faced Zulu woman who asked me many questions about my children. The whole occasion was very memorable and very touching: it was my first experience of this kind, and quite unexpected.)

"It is time to go," Power said now, and as he turned to go I knew that he was about to give me the real reason for his visit: the Bantu are very well-mannered and never rush their messages as we do, falling over ourselves to get them out. "Two days ago my wife saw a little white and black dog running near the house of the school, and at first she thought it just a passing thin dog. But when she looked again she saw that the dog was sick; when she lifted it up, for it was walking very slowly, she saw that it had red marks on his stomach which she thought might be blood. And then she looked again and saw the dog had been sewed up with needle and thread underneath. So she brought it to me and asked, did I not think that this must be a dog that the doctor was treating? – it looks so sick, and has blood and sewing stitches. I said yes to her, perhaps we should ask. Then my wife said that she had heard that you had been sick with the flu, and that we should wait to ask you until you were stronger again. So we tied up the dog and kept it at the school and gave it food. Did we do right, Doctor?"

Power could never have guessed how I felt during that conversation! I was so relieved that I almost burst into tears, and when he brought the dog to me half an hour later – fairly strong and with the stitches still intact, which was amazing – I could not contain myself with joy. "You are wonderful neighbours," I said gratefully, "if Muriel had not seen the dog it would have died. And then the people would have cried, for she is much loved, and I am afraid I would have cried too."

"No, it is the doctor who deserves the thanks, for you have taught us so much about animals and how to take care. If you did not teach us, my wife would have left the dog. My children ask me, how is the grey cat that gave milk to the little black dog?"

"She is strong again, and well, thank you," I replied. "And her little dog child, how is he?"

At that moment Howard arrived, bearing the "little dog child" in his arms, very glad to hear that the post-op stray had been located, especially as he had been one of the people involved in the search. He greeted Power in Zulu, and conversed with him for a few moments until the teacher had to take his leave. "Please, Doctor," he said as he left, "be so kind again and bring the sacks of food for the school in your big van, they will be at the same store tomorrow." Thus we were able to help each other in small ways; his wife taught me Zulu and I helped him with his English; he found my strays and I brought the rations for his pupils. Between us there were no tensions, no difficulties arising out of our varied skin-colour. We were simply parts of the same society, performing our tasks individually as best as we could; the thought of racial strife and resentment did not enter our little world.

Howard Kirk, the farmer-naturalist who had given me my first introduction to the Lowveld's natural heritage, was also my neighbour though his parents' farm lay farther away than the Dzungwes' schoolhouse. Everyone rated as a neighbour in that part of the world provided they were not more than ten miles away! We often rode horses together, visited parks and game-farms, and spent many hours discussing the life and habits of wild life – discussions which were one-sided, for I did all the listening and he did all the instructing.

The Kirk farm was a combination of fertile valleys and hills, a flower, citrus, banana, pineapple and tobacco farm with many side interests, one of which was the glorious shrub- and flower-garden of Howard's petite and lively mother, who kept it beautiful all the year round with the pride and ease of a truly green-fingered gardener. The azaleas, the Bohemias, the dahlias and barberton daisies grew in her domain as they grew nowhere else. She had the gift of decorating her house in such a way as to make her arrangements look as if they were still growing in the fertile earth. Her love and understanding of the soil was equalled only by her son's unique understanding of birds, some of which he kept next to his cottage. They were all waifs and strays, brought to him by the labourers, to whom Howard offered a reward for each one found and brought to him alive. He would nurse an owl with an injured eye, an egret suffering from hail-shock, an infant kingfisher that had fallen from its nest. He usually asked me to help him with these injuries, but I knew that his experience and his touch were far better than mine in this field. His small self-contained cottage, standing some distance away from the main homestead, was a naturalist's haven: he kept there a wonderful collection of books, drawings, slides, journals and above all the photographic equipment which was the most important part of his life, though it was reckoned his hobby. For the rest he worked as a farmer with his father, keeping longer hours than anyone I have ever met. It was he who, in the hour before dawn, rode to the African labourers' compound to wake them for work. When he had finished at night, he did some office work and then plunged into his photographic studies, sometimes getting little or no sleep so that he could catch the hatching of a moth egg, the moulting of a chameleon, or the transformation of a butterfly larva, with his telephoto lens and his arc-lights.

He was quiet and unambitious, his empathy with the wild quite extraordinary. In the bush his shy nature would disappear and he became self-assertive and positive, as alert and keen as the animals which he had made his life's study. In one of his films (set to background music, and with a brief descriptive dialogue) he showed the different types of game quenching their thirst in their varied drinking-places. I tried hard and long to convince my modest friend that his films were world standard, that he need have no compunction about showing them to the public. "They're rubbish," he would say, "I hope I can do better one day." Then one day a professional film-maker, who was a friend of my family, sent word that he had to return to Europe earlier than he had anticipated. Because of cloudy weather, he had been unable to complete his film of Africa: could I help him and find a person who would be willing to sell him some feet of good film? Could I indeed? This was my chance!

As luck would have it, on the night that he came the Kirks had invited some friends to see the very film I loved so much. I took my film-making friend along, and he had grave doubts when I told him that this photographer was actually a full-time farmer. But he did come along, and I watched his face as the film progressed. At the end of the forty minutes I saw him wipe tears from his eyes, as I always did, and sit in silence for a few moments before he spoke. "The uniqueness of your film lies not only in the beautiful photography," he said to Howard, "but in your amazing ability to portray the wild animals as they really are, as they live and move; unhurried, noble, dignified, melting into the earth or the bush, even into their own reflections as they drink." So Howard was launched as a film-maker; and at length he admitted though reluctantly, that some of his sequences were as good as we had maintained.

The puppy that he was now cradling in his arms was Za-Za, foster-child of the cat to which Power had referred. This grey cat had been rescued from under a Pretoria bus by an artist friend of mine; he had given her to me in a state of neglect and enteritis, which had taken me six long months to cure. She grew into an aristocratic-looking queen of a feline, a superlative snake-, rat- and, alas, bird-killer. When a poodle pup had been dumped on my surgery table some months before to be destroyed, I had remembered just in time that Patsy was nursing a new-born litter of kittens and that she might well not object to having one more in her household, even though of a different species. She had needed a little persuasion at first and seemed nonplussed by the furry bundle which neither looked nor smelt like a feline. I finally managed to disguise the pup with some of her own best scent, and after twenty-four hours she accepted the unusual situation with equanimity. The pup had no compunction about accepting a feline mother, and suckled lustily from the very first, pushing her foster brothers and sisters aside as she did so.

After eight weeks the poodle, thoroughbred aristocrat though it was, had adopted a feline attitude and characteristics; she even attempted to mew and move like a cat. She had, by this time, far outgrown her foster family and had taken possession of more than her share of the milk-supply, causing her adopted mother to look very stressed and thin. I then decided to wean her foster-child completely. We had six dogs at that time, four of which were waif-and-stray acquisitions, such as every vet has in abundance and I therefore decided to give the pup to our friends and neighbours, the Kirks, who hitherto had only bred enormous golden ridgebacks. Though at first the men in the Kirk household pretended to have nothing to do with the little bundle, insisting that this diminutive creature could hardly be classed as a dog, they finally succumbed to her charms and eventually became her most ardent admirers. The first months in her new home were fraught with many difficulties; the greatest of these was her partiality to cats. She regarded every cat which crossed her path as a potential milk-bar, and would dive underneath any feline abdomen, male or female, with gusto.

Gradually she came to realise that there was very little to be gained by this behaviour, for she was fiercely repelled by any cat she tackled in that way, and came out of each encounter with little success and many scratches. After some time she resigned herself to the inescapable reality of her breed and began to act like a poodle bitch of the refined variety. Her first litter gave her much joy, and she mothered the three pups most lovingly. The only female of the three was given to us, since at that time our stray community had been thinned out somewhat and we could not resist this little enchantress. We named her Winnie the Pooh, though this name, for the initial months, had a literal and not a literary implication. The cat, Patsy, refused to claim any kinship with the newcomer and would not take on the task of honorary grandmother, preferring the company of the large dogs we kept – one Alsatian and one black labrador. In the end they all curled up together, and when there was an ambulatory patient in the house he or she would join in too. I always had the feeling that in a household such as ours, the animals understood their responsibilities as hosts and hostesses to the visitors; sometimes they even seemed to act as nursemaid or nurse, treating each case differently and with great consideration.

"Is Za-Za sick again?" I now asked Howard, "or have you brought her along just for the visit?" He grinned sheepishly, for his absolute devotion to her was a source of great amusement. "It's her throat again; she cannot swallow without pulling a terrible face. Maybe you will have to take her tonsils out after all." Before I could answer, he had put the dog into my hands and walked out through the hallway and veranda into the garden, listening intently. "Water pump sounds odd," he mumbled, "better go and have a look while you check Za-Za."

While I attended to the poodle with Sam's help, for her mercurial temperament and slippery body kept our hands full, Howard went down to the end of the farm and tinkered with the engine, returning with a happy smile and oily hands long after I had left the surgery. So it had always been; I attended his animals and he looked after my mechanical failures – and there were always many. I was very fortunate in my friends: from the beginning they had helped me with whatever things were beyond my understanding. The inside of a cistern was a mystery to me; and so, to them, was the inside of a horse. Having something which they needed to give in return made life an unending cycle of giving and taking; I often wished that I lived in the days when everything was bartered.

Our friend Bob was the first person we met in the Highlands of the Lowveld, and his kindness meant much to my little family. Our fellowship continued steadily through the years; he had the strange knack of always knowing when we needed something, and always appeared, as if by magic, at the critical time. Too kind, perhaps too concerned for his friends? No, I would answer when that question arose; for never before have I met anyone who gained so much joy from giving and yet who was so gracefully able to receive – not because he really *wanted*, but because he understood that the greatest happiness comes to those who give without seeking anything in return, even a word of thanks.

At this time I also met his brother Theo, master-baker and artist, a happy-go-lucky dynamo, a genius in his own right, dividing his life into periods of isolation (when he would go and paint in far-off lands) and periods of life among people (when he seemed happiest in a crowd of merrymakers or upon the stage of an amateur theatre.) It was as though he needed human contact and a renewed rubbing-up against the core of life, so that he could once again tear himself right away from the mob he so much loved and enjoyed. He was a brave man and one much beloved of his friends, because he was genuine and humorous, and to be with him for a short half-hour would make one feel revived and strengthened. He bore pain so bravely that few knew what he suffered, and this was how he wanted it to be, to the very last; by the time anyone knew that his days were numbered, it was too late.

I once owned a minute Maltese terrier, a stray we named Ricci, for his voice resembled startlingly the sound of the violin of the impresario Ruigeri Ricci, as he tuned it before playing. This amusing, fluffy little dog, the most affectionate one I have ever owned, once entered Theo's studio as he was painting and watched him, his pose at once enchanting, intelligent and inquisitive. Theo captured him on canvas in a few strokes, and came to present me with the portrait which sparkled with skill and with the humour of that white-haired, black-patched, mischievous caricature of a diminutive dog. I shall always remember Theo's black eyes, laughing in his Grecian-type face, his black beard, the darker for the contrast of his pale skin. "It's yours," he said, "maybe one day it will hang in the Royal Academy," and he laughed at his own joke.

In those days when I was just beginning, it mattered greatly to me what people said and thought, for I was unsure of myself, both as a person and as a vet. As the years passed, the importance of people's views lessened, and I relied more upon my sincere friends and upon myself. There was so much that I did not know and could not know; I think that without the help and guidance of the staff at Onderstepoort I would have had many, many more headaches and heartaches. This veterinary institution, the only one in South Africa, was, very fortunately, only two hundred and fifty miles away, and I had the opportunity at the outset to meet many of the staff. They treated me as a colleague and a friend rather than as a stranger from another country and a woman. They endured and tolerated with endless patience my numerous phone calls and appeals for help when I was so often faced with mysteries, or so they seemed to me. Sometimes they could help, sometimes they were baffled too, but always they were polite and friendly. "The Lowveld is disease-stricken, and there is much we cannot tell you about it. Do the best you can, send us specimens, and keep in touch. Remember, if your clients bully you – and they are sure to – we are right behind you: refer to us when you are in trouble, and we will back you up. Remember, we respect you as a fellow veterinarian."

The time I spent at Onderstepoort when I first came to the country stood me in very good stead later. South African diseases had scarcely been touched on in our English curriculum and I had to learn from the beginning in many instances. I knew already of the work that was being carried on at Onderstepoort, for its fame had spread throughout the world and the vaccines produced had saved the lives of countless thousands of animals. I found that the study of African diseases was a tremendous challenge; even then, when the ice of discovery had been broken, they had only touched the fringes of the subject, and while they were carrying on research in one field, a new and hitherto unknown strain of microscopic organisms would begin to wage war against animals and man.

The Lowveld was notorious for its veterinary problems, and the backward state of animal medicine there was partly due to the shortage of vets in the country. Few are prepared to risk the lesser income, the longer hours, the greater wear and tear of country field work; they would rather go from day to day, wading through queues of overfed dogs and cats, living in the smog of cities and wealth rather than brave the uncertainties of the wild but sweet-scented mornings. More and more new graduates have gone into research, or to other countries, or into the remunerative dull life of the towns and cities, unable to fulfil the tradition of the pioneers, unable to take up the challenge of the unknown, ignoring the need of their country whose only hope for economic progress lies in themselves and their own courage.

Very fortunately for me, another veterinarian set up practice, initially by mutual agreement, only fifteen miles away. So after having been alone in this vast area for over a year, I was able at last to take leave without feeling guilty, for this colleague in the valley agreed to do my work while I was away.

Often I tried to time holidays so as to coincide with the veterinary conferences, which are annual occasions. They were well organised, and usually I managed to glean something of real practical interest, apart from being stimulated by contact with vets from every part of the country, and indeed the world. When the veterinary meeting was held in Cape Town for the first time, my friend, Toni Harthoorn – known as 'Darthoorn' among the Zululand rangers, by reason of his unfailing aim with the immobilising gun – was invited to read a paper there dealing with his latest research work on the new synthetic morphine derivative. I decided to take an extra week so that I could first join him in a working trip to Hluhluwe Sanctuary, where there was still much of this work to be done on the white rhinoceros. From there we motored across the breathtakingly spectacular coastal route, known as the Garden Route, one of the loveliest motor trips in the whole of Africa.

This much-needed holiday was a wonderful break; not only did it strengthen me for the coming summer months, always the busiest time, but the rhino-immobilising exercise was one of the most exciting things I have ever seen or done. Above all it brought me once more into close proximity with my old college friend, whom I had previously joined when he was working among antelope and elephant in the Kruger National Park.

On my return, instinct told me more strongly than before that these months of practice – maybe another year – would be my last in the Lowveld. I would never have believed that I could so much enjoy a return to studenthood as in that week in Zululand, carrying instruments and files, learning all I could about this strange new world. I met many devoted and interesting people, such as Ian Player, Chief Conservator of Zululand, whose courage and perserverance and humour have gone a long way to put those sanctuaries on the map, also Gregg Stewart, the first ecologist employed in the Park, and his charming wife. This young man had pitched into the research of the hitherto unknown relationships between the fauna, flora and soil structures of the Reserves, working towards an understanding and maintenance of nature's balance, in spite of man's presence and interference. Then there were Nick Steele, a handsome ranger in charge of the Umfolosi Game Reserve adjoining Hluhluwe, quietly fulfilling his labour of love in the glorious slopes facing the Uvumbo mountains towards the sea; and John Clarke, the hero of the rhinos, father and mother to his beloved charges. I have watched him glowing with pride and love in the *bomas* (enclosures) where the rhinos, newly caught, are gradually tamed; I have even seen him go into the fenced-in strongholds of the very latest arrivals, and the rhinos nuzzle his trouser legs or his always bare feet with obvious pleasure. If any man can grow into a resemblance to wild animals, then John Clarke is that man; he has something of the rhinoceros about him now, though it is hard to know just what it is.

To witness the amazing procedure of immobilisation was the experience of a lifetime. One milligram, one five-hundredth of a standard half-gram M & B tablet, could stop a four-ton rhinoceros within some ten minutes or even sooner. These prehistoric-looking creatures, the 'square-lipped' or white rhinoceros, had not been found in the Transvaal for over a hundred years. They were therefore something of a novelty to me, for one cannot compare a stunted, slow-moving zoo rhino with those I saw in the Reserve in Zululand, free-ranging, heavy, lumbering, tough-skinned moving mountains, their limbs seeming to be artificially jointed to their huge, grey, wrinkled frames.

I watched the first attempt with respect and from a distance, seeing the rhino slow down to a stop, head down, eyes sleepy. I was therefore very surprised when Toni called me to come close and become a rhino-rider! "We want to show the world that a wild rhinoceros can be made safe and still with M99. Would you mind getting on his back for a while so that we can take a photograph?" I was so taken aback that I was tongue-tied and I sleep-walked towards the great beast in a haze, determined not to allow my sex or my lack of courage to hold me back. And soon I was mounted with the aid of someone, I never knew who; to climb on to the peak of a 5,000 lb. mass of flesh, measuring six feet at the shoulder was something I would have thought almost impossible. I hoped that my expression did not show my feelings, but it later proved that I was looking far from confident at the moment when the camera clicked. The rhino was moving slightly, giving me a sensation of sitting high aboard a huge battleship, heaving in the waves.

"It is for the sake of science," my inner voice encouraged me bravely; "do it for science!" "If he really loved you, would he sacrifice you thus?" whispered the fearful, doubting portion of me; "he says he loves you, even wants to marry you; is life, then, going to be one long succession of rhino rides, or maybe worse?" "Promise me," came the remembered warning voice of my mother, "promise me that you will not go near the rhinos; they are even more dangerous than bulls."

"Would you like to come down from your heavenly throne, or do you wish to stay up while we put in the antidote?" This brought me back to reality with a jolt, and down the rhino's back even faster; I had a fleeting vision of being carried through the bush, clinging to the neck of a bucking rhinoceros, unable ever to get off again.

After Zululand, my work seemed a bit of an anticlimax, but I did not mind this as much as I usually did, for I knew that this was my swan-song in practice, and that I was about to embark upon a new period of my life. I would enter this not only as a student, but also happily acquiesce to being a second-class citizeness – a wife, mother and a veterinarian, not in my own right alone, but assisting in a new kind of work, which was holding the world of wild-life conservationists spellbound.

"Are you sure?" my friends asked me. "You have a perfect life here – the work you love, many friends, beautiful scenery, no restrictions, no limitations. Are you certain you want to give up all this for a mere *man*?" Fortunately I could answer with truth that for two years I had felt my days of freedom were coming to an end, and that I had already decided to give up practice before I turned into that image in the formalin bottle, pickled upon the shelf, or much worse into an amazon vet-ess such as my unfortunate party-guest had imagined I must be! I did not realise then that those years of handling animals, of healing, of teaching, of writing, talking and observing, of *living* to the hilt had been years of preparation and no more. I had started off feeling that I could and would conquer the world, that my knowledge was limitless and my skill consummate. The years had at least taught me my own limitations, so that in the end I could know myself still a beginner, ready to start all over again.